THE MIND RESET

Reset Your Mindset, Attain Happiness,

Inner Peace & Grace In Your Life

SARAH JAMES

Book description THE MIND RESET

Do you feel like you should live a happy life? Do you consider yourself weighed down, hindered, and riddled by negative thoughts?

"The Mind Reset" will help you rewire your mindset to see more positive results.

Have you ever wondered why some people get to make their dreams come true, and some people never get anything close to that?

This book will help you learn how to practice positive thinking to make your life a success.

Negative emotions are like standing in a darkened room with a hive of bees. Imagine if you could get light into that room, take advantage of the bees, and attain the honey everywhere!

A positive mind sees more potential and works to your advantage.

Happiness is within the scope of you! Wealthy or poor, regardless of age, whatever your beliefs might be, you should be genuinely happy NOW, not later.

The challenge is that we are reluctant to take risks, to recreate our lives, because we do not understand the mechanism.

This book is realistic and inspiring — full of informative examples that help the reader see that we all face familiar challenges in life but meeting them can be both satisfying and exciting if we equip ourselves with the right resources.

In this guide, we direct our readers through the fundamentals of cultivating happiness in all the facets of life and learn how to use their newly found knowledge to improve the way they feel and behave.

In this book, you will learn:

- How to break the addiction to negative emotions.
- Happiness hacks tailored for each happiness chemical.
- The Attitude of Gratitude.
- Why there is a need to embrace positive thinking.
- The relationship between meditation and spirituality.

Ready to get started? Buy now with 1 click to get your copy of "The Mind Reset" and learn how to increase your happiness and change your mindset today!

website: https://sarahjameslifemastery.com

TABLE OF CONTENTS

INTRODUCTION

Dear friend, is your mind programmed for success or failure? What kind of thoughts? Are they positive most of the time or negative? What is happiness? Is it tangible or invisible? Do these feelings come from your mind, body or soul? These questions and many alike arose in my pursuit for answers. We all want happiness, inner peace, and grace, to find our purpose in this life and leave a vast legacy of humility, before our soul departs into the eternal hereafter.

This book has come into existence, to teach you and me how to live our life. I have sought help from our Creator, The ONE supreme power, to aid me with the best intention to share with you, my experiences and knowledge on how to apply and make our lives valuable.

May we all have a beautiful relationship to please our Creator and to know how to live with the creation in LOVE, LIGHT, and PEACE. No matter what has transpired in our PAST.

I hope you will gain valuable insights and benefits to motivate yourself and others in your life, by applying the actions that resonates with your higher self, leading you effortlessly towards living a meaningful, and purposeful life.

Our happiness is an emotion from within the invisible soul; the superconscious mind is outstanding in its accuracy, perception, and feelings, it resides in the heart close to the solar plexus known as the gut instinct. We are spiritual beings, giving birth to human experiences, either we will evolve, or we will dissolve! We all want to live in a state of harmonious balance, become exemplary role models, and leave a beautiful legacy.

The materialistic World can only induce temporary bursts of happiness, realizing our purpose, results in a deeply satisfying life, regardless of the chaos in our external World.

The ultimate quest for happiness and fulfillment, so, does it exist in our external or internal World?

Deep down, you don't believe in yourself, you are uncertain and insecure about a lot of things.

Are you struggling to communicate effectively with people? Or discover beautiful relationships that are lasting and meaningful? Has your personal life or has your business taken off in the right direction? Have you developed your character? Are you happy, and content with your life?

Are you troubled with procrastination, self-sabotage, impostor syndrome, anxiety, over-analysis, resulting in analysis-paralysis, stress, paranoia, or other symptoms? I can honestly say you are not alone.

It's all deeply buried in your subconscious mind, because you don't believe in yourself. Multiple obstacles arise as a result of the inner stories, you have created in your past, about yourself.

It could be that you believe you are not worthy, or you are afraid of rejection, failure, getting hurt or criticized.

Are others saying you are not good enough or do not deserve to have the best? Have you had your heart broken?

Believe me, I have been there too. Life has been a rollercoaster ride for me, and I have decided never to give up in achieving my dreams for well-being, and heal from the past self-limiting beliefs and post-traumatic experiences.

Do these symptoms make you undervalue yourself, to ask for less than what you deserve? It all has to do with your belief system and lack of trust in God and confidence in yourself.

Our subconscious mind runs 90% of our life.

We all have many limiting, negative and false beliefs within our inner dialogue, most of us have no idea they exist, and these narratives in our minds are the ones that are holding us back.

You need to identify and change them all, to favorable ones to enable you to get rid of all those negative symptoms.

Most people only work on the surface of a problem and do not ever change their personality. Don't be a part of this set of people, discover and unleash your true potential, and authentic self.

Every person in this world would be in a blissful state, if we balance our mindset, with positive thoughts, values and principles.

Money is only an energetic exchange experience of a desire, treat it as such, certainly money plays a vital role in our lives to some degree. In some cases, our happiness is directly proportional to the amount of money we earn and receive. However, we should realize that money, is not synonymous with happiness, and we have heard many times money cannot buy our happiness. Still, we would rather be in a state of gratitude through comfort, security, safety, living abundantly, and being independent, so we may support and provide for ourselves and loved ones.

Marriages are breaking down, parents, children, siblings, extended households are fragmented and dysfunctional, obliterating relations for generations to come. It prevails in all societies, due to the spiritual diseases of the heart, not having heard off or recognizing the existence of these destructive atomic diseases.

Leading to neglect for communication and mutual understanding, appreciation for each other's opinion, self-esteem, confidence, financial accountability, maintaining an agree to disagree strategy, allowing for a peaceful and comfortable life. It's a pandemic, and the impact is tragic to witness people suffering unnecessarily. We are social creatures by nature, and these diseases of the spiritual heart cause destruction to family unity, relationships, and humanity.

The wealthiest people in the World are not necessarily the happiest either! Having witnessed many in my life, the loving, considerate, generous, and the hostile, miserable, offensive people, some are in affluence and others in deprivation. Everyone's state and test is different, wherein they may suffer from unbearable pain, anxiety, stress, depression, fear, sadness, and many additional dilemmas.

We have everything going for us and other times, life is annoying, tragic, and chaotic. We have all witnessed different states in our lives. Every experience is residing within the subconscious part of our mindset. All these various states are invisible, unconscious reactions to our decisions about how we view our internal and external world.

The essence of human senses is such that an emotion is introduced to a specific pleasurable experience, and the perception is continuously exposed to the same sensations. Accordingly, we might not experience pleasure anymore. We get bored or irritated and crave other stimuli. For example, when we eat a favorite meal many times a day, for several days, we begin to dislike the very sight of it. We want to experience something else to get our dopamine surge. The same principle applies to all our senses, with the exception of addictions, such as, smoking, intoxicants, and other stimulants from social media platforms, where people need the urge to hang out to get validation from strangers.

Our World is evolving at a very fast pace, we are constantly exposed to new directions. Engrossed in our worldly pursuits we rarely question, are we on the right path? Is our awareness focused on fulfillment and happiness?

If we reflect within and ask the smart questions, the answers will arrive. Either the teacher will appear when the student is ready to receive, or the answers will come when we seek them out. We will realize that we cannot find lasting satisfaction chasing after material artifacts, happiness is internal, and it does not diminish from the external World.

So, can we ever attain infinite happiness? The answer is yes, we can have happiness in this World and the eternal hereafter, otherwise, what is the purpose of life?

In the eternal hereafter forever, there will never be any ill health and no aging, we will stay eternally youthful, not having to work for a living, no competitions, no futile talks or actions, the cause of harm and suffering from our speech or our hands to any of the creation. The reason for most of the sorrow in this temporary life and no one will have to endure the spiritual illnesses, that we are all suffering from.

All our desires will always get fulfilled, we will receive ever increasing pleasure. There will never be any dissatisfaction whatsoever.

Although right now, in this life we will have to deal with all that we are going to discuss in this book for our mindset, and attitude, that will determine our temporary happiness in this World.

We will encounter waves of happiness for no apparent reason in our lives, so long as we have a plan and execution for all our daily rituals to set the stage for a positive mindset.

Our innate intelligence resides within us, to access it, we must go deep within and do the audit of our inner state. With our breathing, focusing, auto-suggesting, relaxing, all the various parts of our mind-body and soul, and focus on the areas, which will make us feel good and heal us internally and externally.

It is beneficial to do the mind-body, spiritual scanning ritual while lying on your bed or yoga mat. We students are reminded to induce the total mind-body spiritual relaxation technique, at the end of our daily early morning and late afternoon yoga practice, whilst in the corpse pose.

It is an enigma, the illusion of the mindset, raising our vibrational energy with positive thoughts, intentions and words will communicate the same frequency of our vibrational aura.

We must aim for the stars and not ever give up on our dreams, hopes and desires for wellbeing. We should never become despondent or lose hope, as this can interfere with our immunity. If we are prepared to do the mental work, then anything can be achieved. It is our self-imposed limiting beliefs that are the cause of illness and because of our outer circumstances and the change of THE NEW WORLD RESET.

As we are headed into a cashless and digitalized economy, everything is now controlled by the virtual world and monitored.

The media is constantly scaremongering the vulnerable to believe all the fear and uncertainty in the world today, but what is the truth? Is it really a pandemic, or is it an organized ***plan-demic?*** We must all seek the truth and also see the bigger picture because truth and justice will always prevail.

With our inner mindset, with the attitude of grace, love and gratitude, we have the highest and best expectations from our Creator, after all he is the knower of the unseen truth.

He helps us see our truth and achieve whatever we desire to help facilitate us in our life, everything is a blessing in disguise, even though it may not seem so, the one on truth and seeker of the divine will be guided.

In God we put our faith and trust as he says ***"I am as my servant thinks of me"*** He has created this World to test us between the forces of good and evil.

We can choose to think the thoughts that will make us feel peaceful and happy. All our wishes, dreams and desires will manifest, what is right that feels good is always available, and so is what is wrong. We have a choice to decide how, we will think and feel, in any given moment in our life.

Do you crave for optimal health, comfort, luxury, wealth, beauty, happiness, a peaceful life? What about your relationship with the

Creator, the creation, and the preparation for the eternal hereafter? Yes? Good, you can have it all, affirm, believe, seek beneficial knowledge, practice till you make perfect, apply the proficiency into action, meditate and pray every day. It will become a reality sooner than you think. I have seen it in my own life. Reset the story of your life in your mindset first, change your attitude and willingly participate.

We furthermore must be very mindful, guard the door of our mind and outside influences, that way we can realize that our negative thoughts, emotions, and actions hold us back from achieving profound happiness. To have peace of mind; we need to become free from the negativity that plagues us all.

The spiritual diseases of the heart is an invisible disease that manifests negative feelings and triggers reactions, such as selfishness, greed, arrogance, aggression, anger, jealousy, hatred, malice, resentment, instability, violence, corruption, oppression, misguidance, betrayal, transgression, violating the rights of the Creator and his creation.

Extensively worse symptoms arise if not dealt with. The list is almost endless, which is an extra reason to guard ourselves against such unpleasant emotions; the worse our mental state is, the more negative emotions will transpire. —Infusing more power to these emotional discomforts is a sure setup for more failures. It becomes a facet of life, a vicious sequence unless it is eradicated out of one's existence.

Many of us need guidance towards healing ourselves; the final holy scripture, the Noble Quran, the most beautiful LOVE letter from GOD to humanity, shows us direction on how to heal and live our life. His chosen spiritual Prophets, the sages, masters, and experts throughout history inform us, we have caused oppression on our souls.

I am sure you have identified some of these facets in your life. Either we reflect them and are not aware of their existence, or we have learned these mirrored patterns from others, and we have not acknowledged they reside within us.

Whichever option it is, none of us are exempt; these behaviors are learned from our ancestors and absorbed during our infancy. The good news is, they can all be erased by rewiring our thoughts, emotions, and actions.

We are, and become the company we associate, and what we intake to nourish our physical bodies, as we have all heard many times, we are what we eat. I have referred to a few of the over excess imbalances, described in the chakra system, as they are all corresponding and they affect us, spiritually, mentally, physically, emotionally, and psychologically.

Looking at the big picture, we want to be free of these spiritual diseases, the first step is becoming aware and recognizing these characteristics, then we must eradicate them out of our life one by one. Through self-development, we all have different degrees, some are very acute spiritual diseases of the heart. If our heart is in darkness, how can light enter?

Look at the soul as the driver and the physical body as the vehicle, just as the body needs nourishment, from food and drink, the soul needs nourishment, from the remembrance of our Creator.

The subject of the spiritual heart and its cures is a very vast topic and deserves to be covered in its own entirety, which will be conveyed in the sequels for advice to achieving happiness to "The Mind Reset." I hope you gain value and enjoy reading my books or listening to them on audios and applying in your life and see the changes happen in your life with grace and effortless ease.

The thoughts we think and the emotions we feel in any present moment will sow the seeds to grow into our mental state. Our conditioned mind and subconscious minds, have had experiences which have left an imprint on us, so it is up to us to rewire our mindset to eliminate the negative thought patterns.

Let us get to the root cause, and really take a deep dive, we must understand now, and rewire our mindset so we can set a solid foundation for a happy and successful life.

In this modern day, we get so distracted, we can sometimes forget about the important things that matter. All the chaos, worries, anxieties, etc. are the cause of the toxic chronic pains and ill health we suffer in the physical body. It is very difficult for many people to experience inner peace, joy, and satisfaction, when burdened with chronic mental and physical pain.

You see we need to change our dialogue when we are in pain and suffering, and really focus our attention on some deep breathing, taking a few minutes to become present. Let go of what does not serve us, with optimistic thoughts, statements, prayers, and meditative states.

I am here to offer you a blueprint from my own life experiences. The mentors and teachers who appeared in my life to help me with my healing, insights and wisdom. It is my commitment to enhance my own life's work that is in progress every day, to make a difference in my life and the lives of others.

We must intend to help and serve the creation, in which ever path we can. The hormone oxytocin is released when we serve or give without any expectation; the giver feels the expansion of joy and happiness from within the soul. We must understand the creation is a test for us, and we are a test for the creation.

I start my book off with a prayer for ***"All Seekers Of Truth."***

"Oh you, who has created us, show us truth and help us towards it, show us falsehood, and help us to avoid it. Comfort and enlighten us to a peaceful, happy life in both worlds. Bless us with your love, and the way of life which you love, and make everything beautiful and easy for us."

It is all a reminder for me first and foremost to put into practice all that I have reflected in the book and to remind my readers that we will all gain priceless insights and wisdom. We are the 100% beneficiaries and the value in this book is to serve as a reminder to help reset our mindset, enhance our happiness, inner peace, divine love, tranquillity, and serenity in our life, regardless of all the turbulence and illusions in our external world, and may it lead us all to the assured success and salvation in our everlasting hereafter. Amen.

CHAPTER 1
THE POWER OF THE MIND

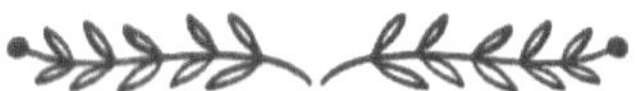

"Your mind is a powerful tool. When you fill it with positive thoughts, your life will start to change."

Imagination power is amongst the most potent and valuable abilities you have. The power of the mind can build successes and failures, joy or displeasure, openings or challenges, together with your imagination, and that is up to your attitude.

The major component of this force is your thoughts, and when you add concentration, emotion and feelings arising to them, our thoughts bring energy so strong they can influence our words, actions, habits, character, and our destiny.

Not every single thought is equivalent. Stray thoughts you think once or twice will not affect you, but your prevailing thoughts, stories, and opinions will influence your attitude, personality, and actions. These prevailing thoughts will have an affect on your life experiences.

In our quest for progress, more innovation, accomplishments, and many other personal development manifestations, there are unique components of the mind that can be used to enhance our growth exponentially. When we talk about the reason, it's essential to realize that our total mind is composed of three independent parts that when used together adequately, we can virtually ensure success in all areas of our life.

The conscious, subconscious, and superconscious are the crucial components that make up the whole mind, and the favorite aspect is that we all have these incredible resources centralized in our mind, body and soul!

Each of the facets of the mind is a critical element, crafted by our Creator to help us fulfill our wishes, aspirations, and desires.

As we pay closer attention to our inner dialogue, we will appreciate, our mind serves as the united front of the conscious, subconscious, and the superconscious intelligence. Let us take a more in-depth look at all three levels of consciousness, so that we can fully comprehend how our mind operates.

Understanding The Relationship Between The Conscious, Subconscious & The Superconscious Mind

The conscious mind can be perceived as the machine function of the mind. It does have a unique role to play by providing us safety.

Let us look at how it operates in collaboration with the other two components of the mind to realize the observations and knowledge that comes to us to understated, barely visible signals.

When talking about the influence of the conscious mind, the conscious mind is responsible for our actions, while the subconscious mind takes charge of the reactions, and these reactions are as significant as the actions.

Based on this premise, most people believe, that our conscious mind determines our personality. In reality, however, our conscious mind is only a minor fraction of who we are. It's a tiny fraction of how the three components of our mind allow us to interact with the world.

Even though our conscious mind is readily available, that doesn't mean it's the instrument that decides our personality, our actions, and the reasons behind our actions. It is a medium that allows us to communicate efficiently through our words, images, writings, physical acts, and our limited thought mode.

The Role Of The Conscious Mind

The conscious mind is our rational mind. It doesn't have a memory, and it can only carry a single thought at a time. It is used to organize new messages through our senses of feeling, sound, sight, smell, touch, and taste.

Our conscious mind keeps analyzing and classifying (accurately or innacurately) what happens around us. It is the section of our mind that can't be trusted entirely.

It is always sorting through our thoughts; analyzing our experiences to ultimately determine which ones are important and which are not.

The subconscious mind is also affected by our past behavior and previously incorrect decisions, it is like a binary machine. It supports or refuses issues in a straightforward "yes" or "no" manner to decide about something. It deals with one thing at a time: positive or negative.

The advantage of this sort of philosophy is that the conscious mind makes sure the safety and security of our lives. It helps us to decide quickly on issues. Our subconscious, on the other hand, is like a vast memory archive. It's capacity is practically infinite and stores all that has ever happened to us permanently.

Now that you understand how the conscious mind functions, let's take a more in-depth look at the subconscious mind, it's purpose in our lives and its relationship with intuition.

In discovering the degree that resides at the base of our conscious mind, we come to the subconscious mind. It's the part of our mind that tracks all our actions and thoughts, the feelings we have about those activities, and the preferences we experience each day. It is the portion of our mind that still works while we are asleep, dreaming, and acting according to the values that we do not know approximately.

While the subconscious mind overlooks nothing, this portion of our intellect remains concealed from our daily consciousness. However, that does not exempt it from affecting how we think and behave in our state of awareness.

In other words, the subconscious affects much of our actions every day, but those effects come from previous behavior and the patterns that we have developed from them. This means that the thoughts generated from the subconscious mind is not fresh and imaginative.

Our subconscious mind gives meaning to all of our experiences that is assuming it is interpreted through our values and personality.

How The Subconscious Mind Functions

The subconscious mind expresses knowledge through our thoughts, desires, visions, perceptions and dreams. Our present perception of consciousness is static. It fails to understand conscious events beyond the concept of real. Such events are known to be fraudulent, abnormal, or unusual.

Your consciousness is connected to the world and is only natural in the sense that it is well-known; you are aware of everything on the outside as well as specific basic cognitive processes occurring in our intellect.

It is pertinent to realize that your subconscious mind cannot step outside its established norms – it responds automatically to circumstances in a pre-stored behavioral response. It operates without the awareness or control of the mind. That is why we are sometimes so unaware of our actions.

Studies from as far back as the 1970s suggest that our brains begin to plan an action 0.2-sec ahead before we actively decide to act. In other words, even though we 'think' we are awake, it is our subconscious mind that is responsible for our decision-making system.

When you go into reflection or prayers, and you start regulating your breathing, you will get power from the subconscious mind and transfer into your conscious mind.

Inhale deeply and exhale entirely then stop regulating the breath and your subconscious mind takes over. You no longer need to be concerned, your breathing will continue to calm until it transitions to another stimuli, for example anxiety or stress. Everything is controlled and running in the background of your subconscious illumination.

The conscious mind is about thinking, analyzing and storing short-term memory inside the brain. It generates images and regulates the 'force of will' through your senses, it is in contact with your surroundings. During the waking state, it is mainly in control of your consciousness (awareness).

On the other hand, the subconscious mind is non-judgmental. It neither knows logic nor does it performs any analysis. It pretty much submits to conscious mind rules. It holds a gigantic long-term memory store, to which it adds every new knowledge that the conscious mind receives.

The subconscious mind runs all day and takes care of your consciousness while you sleep. It's accessible until dulled by the conscious mind and the senses. The subconscious mind is accountable for all the necessary actions carried out by the body's internal organs such as heart rate, lung activity, digestion, etc. It also takes care of automatic pilot tasks, for example, while driving a vehicle.

It is significant to comprehend the subconscious mind registers only the 'good' version of knowledge that the conscious mind transmits. In other words, it does not accept terms such as "not," "wouldn't," "don't," etc. For instance, if your conscious mind says, "I am not bad" during the inner dialogue, The subconscious mind will record "I am bad," If you say "I will not fail," it will record "I will fail."

This is how God has fashioned our minds. The more you get to understand how your mind works and accept it's functioning, the more you will have power over it.

The subconscious mind is your behavior storage facility, it records all your actions, thoughts, and feelings from infancy and all your waking life experiences. And what happens with the information obtained from the conscious mind by the subconscious mind. You may not like this, but the subconscious mind operates on the theory of "If you tell me, I'm going to tell God" and it doesn't matter what it is, every intention, thought, word, and action is recorded, transparent and transmits as a vibrational frequency.

The fundamental mind works relentlessly to develop real-life alternatives of your earthly empathic waves for you. You may not see the self assurance, but in a matter of time, you will see it as definitely as the morning comes after the night.

If you have any understanding of factory work, you can think of converting your emotional vibrations into look-alike molds as they enter the metaphysical domain. They arrive on God's assembly line, and Divine intellect infuses them with the substance that produces exact copies of your emotions in real life. Then the Divine mail carrier sends you the manufactured items in the form of 'characterized situations in your life.' And oh, "rates of return are not accepted"- the products will not arrive anyway with an address to return!

The conscious mind is connected to the subconscious mind as a model, and the subconscious mind is connected to the Superconscious Mind.

Only one Superconscious mind exists, linked to your subconscious mind, the proportion of the superconscious mind is what is often called the Higher Self. This is the Sacred Light that is pure within your soul that you came with when you were born, but it gets tarnished and goes into darkness and these spiritual diseases form so we want a cure for these spiritual diseases of the soul.

The Higher Consciousness of all beings is bound together to create a Superconscious mind. It is from the Superconscious mind that our God-like attributes come from: for example the names of God are he loves us more than all the mothers he has created, so, we must love, just as a mother has natural instinct to love and protect her child, he is the most Beautiful, we are excessively attracted to beauty, and also want to look and feel beautiful, he is the most Merciful, we show mercy to his creation, he loves to Forgive his creation, we must also get into the habit of forgiving and repenting, he is so Compassionate, we must show compassion to all his creation, he is Kind and Generous, we must show acts of kindness and generosity, he is the Divine Creator, we also have unique divine creative expressions within us, he is all encompassing etc, he has names that we know of and many other names we do not know of, he has created mankind and bestowed upon us the most elevated status of all his creations.

The names of God are in his attributes, the Superconscious mind is connected to the mind of God, we are not separate from him, he is the all knowing, he sees us, he hears us, and he is all around us, he knows what is in the hearts of all his creation, we can inquire and acquire, at the very least the noble subtle qualities within the names of God, he is ONE and unique, he does not resemble the creation, he is unlike any of his creation and more beautiful than anything he has created, without any partners or deities, we are his creation, we confide and trust in him, we are created for the sole purpose of worshipping him alone, his mercy outweighs his wrath, so we have hope in his mercy, for our entire life and eternal hereafter is dependant on his mercy, and we can turn to him to help us with anything, everything is possible and nothing is impossible for him, it is our beliefs that set up the limitations or expansion in our life.

We can never be perfect as God is perfect and we are imperfect beings, but we must aim for advancement and constantly raise our standards, and we do the very best we can and leave the rest to our Creator, as we are only the creation and dependant on him for everything in existance. The millions of universes are his creation and there are many worlds and universes and entities that he has created that are in parallel existence to our world, that we don't know anything about in the infinite vast space. Everything is under his universal laws, are in cause and effect, and under his order to serve his commands. We can't lift a finger without his permission and neither can the leaf fall off a tree without his command.

Why do people ask for things from the universe? He established the cosmos, to administer his command, so we must go directly to him and ask whatever we desire from the Source.

It is incredibly comforting to turn to him anytime we need him, he is the only ONE who adores us, he loves to listen and dispense unto us, the creation is not always tolerant, as some will get impatient and frustrated with us at times if we seek out their help.

God, "oh my" he is so kind, loving, and tolerant, he is pleased and happy to help us, to rescue us at any time we seek his help, the universe is created to serve his creation in the invisible unseen World.

His angels are created from light and they do not have any free will, they are pure, innocent entities, they only do good, as commanded by God. We have angels all around us guiding and protecting us; there are more angels created than humans, they inspire us to think good thoughts, impulses are sent into our minds and hearts to feel good emotions and perform good actions.

And there is the devil satan, he is the outcast, he is created out of smokeless fire, he is our enemy, the mischief troublemaker, he is arrogant and jealous of us, he whispers suspicious, evil thoughts, into humanity. Then we trip up, we fall for his trap big time, we think these are our thoughts, he makes everything so alluring, he dares to convince us that wrongdoing is not evil or bad, it's so critical now, we have to be so alert and be on our guard, he will destroy us if we allow his evil to permeate our mind-body and soul!

Whether you believe or not this is the truth, so the purpose of our life is to rid us of the malady of the spiritual diseases of the heart, before our very limited time on Earth ends, this eternal soul must become a shining sound heart, before it goes back to God, to live eternally in the hereafter, the most beautiful sight we want is the perfect vision of God, this is the ultimate accomplishment for our permanent life in the hereafter. We will only be able to comprehend, when we see him and nothing will be in comparison to his magnificence not in any of his creation.

"Surely we belong to him and surely our return is back to him," he wants our eternal soul back to him, the way he gave us our pure untarnished soul, which existed in the world of souls, before it arrived to live on Earth.

Have you ever thought about why we are here and what is our purpose in the temporary World?

The conscious mind contacts the subconscious mind with its thoughts and emotions. In turn, the conscious mind collects knowledge from the subconscious mind on long-term memory during moments of recollection.

The conscious mind may also obtain hunches and inspirations from the subconscious mind in the form of thoughts, visual images, or the well-known 'inner voice' when the conditions are right.

As regards, the superconscious mind is ever exciting yet complex, superconsciousness is a dimension of its own. This is level three and beyond of the mind that directs us in our path in life.

While we are quite familiar with the conscious and the subconscious mind, still the superconscious mind remains elusive and ambiguous to many due to lack of belief, just because science has not been able to transmit enough proof.

It is the ancient belief structure of insight for prayers, miracles, meditation, physical, moral healing, seeking guidance, truth and goodness. It's a problem-solving part of us, and it helps us experience things like joy, enthusiasm, and compassion. Our superconscious mind's role is often ignored as we aspire for a better, more worthwhile life.

Although we are acquainted with brief moments of heightened awareness, only few know how to deliberately access the exalted state of superconsciousness.

Superconsciousness is a condition that can only be achieved by meditation, vibration of sound, true sincere belief, and prayers, explicitly designed to bring us to a condition of superconsciousness. It is the superconscious mind that makes it possible for human beings to achieve perfection and raise the human spirit.

The idea is premised on reaching our higher self, which encompasses reality. It is the nature of human life that makes us capable of moving beyond the physical realm's limits, the distinction and circumstance of rationality.

The relationship between the subconscious mind and the superconscious mind is often bi-directional. Forward the subconscious mind, vibratory patterns of stimuli obtained from the conscious mind to the superconscious mind. The superconscious mind transfers intuitions and ideas to the subconscious mind in the backward pass, to be forwarded to the conscious mind when the necessary conditions are formed within the individual.

"Keep on the fire" don't get the jitters. It is your dominant thoughts and emotions that manifest in your life and there are ways of gaining power over them. Look at the bright side, this is a phenomenal opportunity for you to influence your destiny!

Reprogramming Your Subconscious Mind

The subconscious mind unconsciously influences our thoughts and behavior by the programming instructions or language through which it works. This is generated by our database of accumulated values, life experiences, and impressions of the world around us. We can actively re-write our subconscious thoughts, acquiring more power over our lives through advanced practice.

Why Reprogram The Subconscious?

Considering and appreciating this large, healthy, and significant portion of our mind, most of us will prefer a life that expands continuously in a positive way, benefiting us personally and as a natural by-product, the well-being of others. If this admirable desire is understood in a practical sense, the consequences for improving all of life would inevitably be profound, as we become implicitly connected.

By cohesively linking the two minds in a meaningful manner and understanding their experiences, we may begin reprogramming parts of our subconscious mind, which are liable for self-sabotaging our real, highest aspirations and wishes. In the natural, every day life course, we experience repetitive but seemingly secret symptoms stored in our subconscious that hinder typically displayed pleasure, efficiency, achievement, and healthy living, sharing our highest intent. At this stage, consciousness emerges, and we begin to understand that something is influencing our actions and resolving to address these contradictions within us with the best expectations.

This is a turning point full of fantastic opportunities! The best examples of these deeply concealed symptoms produced by the subconscious are those with a significant emotional power *"signature of a memory."*

However, one example stored is feeling a dismissal from somebody you cared for or love. In the following situation involving a presumed possibility for rejection, our conscious mind will rapidly obtain an implicit subconscious interference to explain why rejection will occur. While this is a flawed belief, you might unknowingly be the one to sabotage in advance, the chance that another person or circumstance might wish to experience maximum acceptance. The same applies to intense, emotionally charged low self-esteem disputes, that occurred whenever you encountered feelings of inadequacy, perceived failure, or when someone suggested or labelled you with incompetence, worthlessness or undesirable names etc.

The negative taunts or connotations exude powerful imagery, that can lead to a prolonged period of suffering in many aspects of your life, unless it is reversed or eliminated from your subconscious makeup. It is not so difficult to reprogram your subconscious to combat the negatively charged embedded responses, if you can follow a few necessary procedures, that will significantly enhance your mental health and external reaction to life as a whole over time.

Reprogramming Checkup List

Here are 17 points of light that are typical to note, ponder, and apply while causing desired changes to your subconscious. This is truly a lifestyle and noble endeavor that provides rich rewards both individually and in the larger world around you. Below are some well-known and less well-known thoughts and acts that are easily implemented to help you promote a better, improved you! Find what resonates with you while evaluating the list, and note what those feelings are (no matter positive or negative). This feeling-based approach will give you useful, emotionally driven insights into those things that will change your life as quickly as possible when implemented. Your most important guideline is always your greatest good, that little voice never leads you astray. Recognize this moral vital, more impartial direction and reap incredible changes in every aspect of life. Like they say- It is nice to take daily checkups from the neck up.

1. Before anything, believe in yourself.

2. Identify and describe what holds you back, so that you can conquer it.

3. Spend time every day in peaceful self-reflection, prayer, and meditation.

4. Still, your mind, be the observer of the thoughts without any judgment, and become the witness.

5. Know, in exact words, what you want.

6. Eradicate from your life all causes of negative mind chatter.

7. Surround yourself with optimistic people who are already where, you want to be.

8. Build a concrete strategy to make your greatest dreams come true.

9. Every day, take constructive measures towards your plans and visions in life.

10. Focus on the present moment-as if the things you want are already here with you.

11. Build visual boards and reminders of your thoughts and priorities.

12. Record your favorite affirmations and listen to them daily or rehearse them.

13. Prevent inner disputes which can trigger your emotions as they could manifest.

14. Write in your journal of your success as if it has happened already.

15. Be a self-advocate, allowing for appreciation and feedback.

16. I always want the right outlook and a positive mentality.

17. I want the experience of an extraordinary life, and I envision it every day.

The Role Of Your Conscious Mind

First of all, recognize and appreciate yourself for reading thus far as this is a mental discipline testimony and a desire to become a more awake human being. Together we are all on this journey, so be careful with all this and be easy on yourself—Avoid self-perception-beating, which sometimes precedes any challenge to undesirable conditioned responses generated by the subconscious self-importance.

Knowing this whole phase is not that difficult, and some bull-headed character traits you want to change can take time to saturate your subconscious for the better.

Just decide to participate enthusiastically and start the process. And not to be overlooked, as we have eternity to achieve a high state of vibration even if it isn't perfect, fake it till you make it!

You have to learn to use your mental powers, practice your own mind's effectiveness. It requires the belief of possibilities and getting rid of the confusions and pressures of our everyday lives.

Practicing meditation is very helpful, allowing the mind to concentrate on the breathing and making an intention, the mercy of God is falling on your heart, a pure divine light is raining down into your heart and it is your heart chanting the beautiful name of God and you are the observer and becoming the witnessed, this is a very powerful meditation, the hearts find rest in the remembrance of God, it is easy and simple, I was taught this profound and powerful meditation from my beloved, spiritual guide and teacher who now resides in the UAE, it is the cure for the spiritual diseases of the soul and makes the spiritual heart sound and polished to sparkle like a diamond, so light may enter, making the soul purified so it can distinguish right that will benefit and the wrong that can harm and destroy the spirit.

Meditation simply frees yourself, especially your mind, from all the worries and stressful thoughts, in turn think of happy memories, appreciate those moments and feel gratitude, for when you are grateful you can't be stressed or angry simultaneously. This will allow the conscious and the subconscious mind to rest, While meditation has many strategies and basics, it would be better for beginners to stick to the most convenient or appropriate approach for your lifestyle, the object is to attain inner peace and stillness, you can start modeling the mind's widely accessible resources to get what you want. It may be difficult at first, but you will realize that it's not that difficult through proper guidance and a strong desire to accomplish your dreams and ambitions.

You will start learning the power of the mind to imagine its purpose after practicing meditation. You want to be abundantly rich, for example, after reflecting on that target and having a deep desire to achieve that dream, start visualizing yourself inside the house of your dreams, driving the most luxurious and latest transportation or model sports car, investing thousands of dollars for investing for your future, travelling and shopping in one month or serving noble causes and charities, feel the sensations, breath and feel, it is all real and here in the present moment now, as if you are already living it. These will incentivize you to work towards your desires to make those wishes a reality.

The subconscious mind does not know, that what you are thinking or affirming in the present tense has not arrived yet, it will take for real whatever it is you desire and it is very real to the subconscious mind. You can also encourage others to pursue what you find valuable, by using the mind's forces, to create a better life for you and your significant others. In the end, everything depends on your willpower, as you will have to do the work to translate your mind's power to get to where you want to be.

Accessing Your Superconscious Mind

The theories behind the superconscious state of mind are genius-level insight, inspiring intuition, a surprising flow of thoughts, motivation, and excitement. We will have access to the "higher self" the superconscious side to understand the world.

The superconscious mind, also recognized as the higher-self can be accessed through meditation. The person should practice keeping the spine straight, guiding your energy to the superconsciousness seat between the eyebrows, also known as the inner third eye Ajna chakra. Genuine intuition and healing can happen at this stage, for example, through the practice of positive intentions and devotion.

When we tap into the superconscious mind, we go beyond our physical bodies and into the celestial realms. In reality, the superconscious mind is referred to by many as the soul, or universal consciousness. Our souls have extraordinary forces and relations that go far beyond our physical world.

Because of the universal mind's unique connection to all other minds and limitless wisdom, many psychic powers are possible when we practice our superconsciousness, which makes some of the incredible supernatural abilities open to those who understand how to tap into the superconscious mind's energies.

Together with the exceptional psychic powers intrinsic in all of us, being tuned into the collective psyche gives us the ability to unlock the enormous volume of information that is part of the superconscious mind. Many names have been given to this vast knowledge base all across history, and incredibly, this comprehensive database is obtainable to anybody who learns how to leverage it.

Concerning the overall success of our desires, the superconscious mind can be actively involved in bringing into our lives specific opportunities and synchronicities that can help speed up our dreams and goals. In combination with our subconscious minds and acceptable behaviours, it helps develop our superconscious minds work in the metaphysical realms to make our hopes and dreams come true.

Access To The Lower Levels Of Superconsciousness

We will delve into the lower ranks of superconsciousness. First, the superconscious mind is your imagination, brilliant thoughts, higher-self, mind-flow, heart consciousness, and limitless intelligence.

There are seven that intensify the effects and make it easier to reach superconscious frequencies.

Note, this practice takes time and consistency is the key. The rewards are well worth the effort and time.

1. Get into the states of love, appreciation and gratitude, is the highest frequency, feel your passion; feel your gratitude. It's not enough to think about it, feel it and believe it.

2. Breathing and moving is nature's cure, a flexible body makes a flexible mind.

   Run, walk, dance, swim, practice yoga, qigong, tai chi, pilates, or cycling, anything to enhance your breath control, keep your body safe and supple. A static body can impede energy flow and can also trigger stress or pain.

3. Relax the body, mind and soul and go with the flow of life, just as the tree branches flow wherever the wind gives her direction.

   It would help if you relaxed for energy to flow into the body. You can speak to the practitioners of Yoga and Qigong. They are going to agree.

4. Ask and decide what you want in your life. Set your goal. Adapt your mental resources to the desired result.

5. When your genius-level thought and creativity arrive, do not doubt it, don't ruin your life with rational, theoretical, or critical thinking. Ensure that you allow it to flow through you, feeling deserving of it and confident in it.

6. Eat clean, eat for vibration.

To maintain states of high vibrations, you want to keep your body healthy, eat foods that boosts your states of high vibration, nourishing wholesome organic food, prepare the food yourself, pray whilst preparing your food, and no processed or prepackaged foods.

This allows your body, the energy vessel, to retain these higher frequencies better. Fasting is a great booster that helps the body to shift through higher vibrations.

7. Mindfulness meditation practice. When you begin mindfulness meditation for the first time, you begin to tap into the Super consciousness. If you continue to practice meditation and mindfulness, you will finally feel the 'split' of an enhanced degree of consciousness that surpasses your relationship with yourself and your body. And you're feeling universal, super, or harmony consciousness.

Conclusively, the self realizes that superconsciousness is the truth of being compared to disrupted states of our awareness. Then being constrained by conscious thinking or subconscious emotions, the mind is liberated from captivity.

The flow state is beyond the superconscious. A form of being where you are mentally focused and accessible. Otherwise, it is known as *"being in the woods."* If we have a perfect meditation and feel *"absolute calm and centeredness,"* we start to reach a degree of superconsciousness. When we go deeper into meditation and encounter more profound harmony, serenity, divine love, and even happiness, we get deeper layers of the superconscious. Einstein described this as the *"mystical emotion"* – the slightest emotion we are capable of. I call it a state of *"blissful ecstasy!"*

CHAPTER 2
TAKE CHARGE OF YOUR THOUGHTS

"Bad news is that you can control nothing but your thoughts. Good news is that with your thoughts you can control everything else."

Are you pleased with your life? The question itself is full of sense and most of us would offer mixed answers if we were truthful. Most of life is made up of different situations, in which we are happy with certain parts of life and unhappy with others. As tempting as it is to rely on a change in circumstances to find satisfaction in life, the fact is that your attitude dictates your happiness, not your circumstances. So learning how to control your mind is key to creating a sense of serenity with yourself and your life, whatever the circumstances. When you know how to take control of your mind, you will find balanced contentment.

Knowing how to control your mind starts by understanding that you are in complete control of your body. Since your mind, body, and emotions are interlinked, you can use mind-body strategies to bring you greater knowledge to your thought, which affects your feelings. When you accept the practice of living in the moment, you become more adept at retaining self-awareness in any situation, Tony Robbins says, it is the practice of accepting self-awareness in the present moment that ultimately drives long-lasting happiness and contentment.

In reality, self-determination research shows that the more you believe you are in charge of your circumstances (by remaining grounded in the moment), the more productive and happy you are likely to be. Around this time, avoid the temptation to take a "TGIF" approach on life and only live for the weekend (or whatever high points you choose to prioritize over more mundane dull moments of your life). Instead of wishing you will only be happy when you arrive at the destination, accept your current life, enjoy the journey whilst you are in the process to get to your desired destination in life and you will be on your way to understanding and managing your philosophy.

Can We Control Our Thoughts?

Wouldn't it be awesome if we had just thoughts and emotions that we liked and needed and could erase the rest? I would love it, if any idea or feeling came into my mind, came within my logical, natural, and healthy concept. What a victory that would have been a mental perfection that I've always wanted. I don't think I'm alone in wishing that my mind was like an exact greenhouse, a place where only reassuring, productive, politically correct, and good thoughts arose. Many people wish they do not have to deal with things like, "I don't want to worry about this anymore," or, "I want to stop having those feelings."

These realistic goals can often mask a hidden quest for self-perfection: ***"I want to purify my mind from things that I find to be unreasonable, evil, or sick."*** We want our crazy thoughts out and our "safe," civilized, "good" ideas to govern. And there's nothing wrong with hoping for that.

When we follow this idea and attempt to make it a fact, however, we seek an unrealistic illusion of undeniably perfect control; we forget that while we seem to be highly civilized creatures, we are still creatures with automatic, uncontrollable facets of our minds and nerves. We forget that while we are now physically adults, we were once children. We emulate a legacy of childlike emotions, feelings, and memories that we can never fully outgrow or forget.

Unfortunately, often we are faced with the impossible: to obtain complete control of the brain, which depends almost entirely on unconscious, automatic, unregulated processing. When we do this and ask therapists to join us in this mission, what will happen to us and our therapy? Will we learn to live with a mind that can generate logical and "wild" thoughts? Have we got a choice?

We are aware of a small portion of the thinking that is going on in our minds, and we can control only a tiny part of our cognitive thoughts. The overwhelming majority of our thought and activities go on subconsciously. Only one or two of these thoughts are likely to come into awareness at a time. Slips of the tongue and involuntary acts offer a snapshot into our unfiltered, subconscious mental reality.

The unwanted thoughts that one might have experienced in the day or before bed illustrate the disturbing fact that many of the mind's functions are beyond conscious control. The central debate on free will is whether we retain proper control over any mental process. Maybe this loss of control is to be assumed as the basis for almost all the mind's labors have been laid long before the consciousness of our ancestors, evolution.

Even intentional decisions are not entirely within our power. Our awareness only sets the start and the end of the objective but leaves unconscious mental processes. As a result, for example, a batter can decide to swing at a ball, that enters the strike zone and demarcate that zone's borders. But when the balls pass through, the mental functions of the unconscious take over. The intentions required to send the batter to the first base are too complicated and too quick to maintain our slow, conscious influence.

We exercise some control over our thoughts by focusing our attention, like a spotlight, to concentrate on something important. The effects of doing so can be funny, as in the recent tests in which about one-third of the people watching a basketball game were unable to spot a man in a gorilla suit across the court. Or the effects can be catastrophic, as if a narrow focus prevents a driver from seeing a red light or an oncoming train.

Though our thoughts tend to "pop" into consciousness before bedtime, their cognitive precursors have probably been simmering for a while. If those preconscious thoughts collect enough power, the full light of consciousness shines down upon them, so the mind's free-wheeling, friskiness is only partially under our control, so turning our minds off until we sleep is difficult.

- What controls your mind and the thoughts that run in it?
- Are you able to determine which thoughts to consider and which ones to reject?

What about other people's thoughts, the ideas and opinions of the people you meet, and the suggestions and knowledge you get from the TV or the Internet and social media? Can they influence your attention? Yes they sure do.

Most people do not understand all the thoughts that flow through their head, since most thinking is done unconsciously.

Most often, the mind behaves like an innocent child, who embraces and takes for truth granted whatever he sees or hears, without judgment or without considering the implications. If you let your mind function in this way, you lose your freedom.

We are continuously bombarded with opinions, debates, views, suggestions, and information from the five senses, the people in our lives, the TV, internet, youtube, newspapers, books and social media. These thoughts, ideas and knowledge enter the mind and influence our behavior and state of mind, whether or not we are conscious of this process.

This flow of thought influences our personality and reactions. It affects the way we think, our tastes, likes and dislikes. Typically, we immediately embrace these feelings, allowing them to form our lives. In reality, this means that we lose the freedom of our mind.

The Source Of Your Thoughts

Do you believe and think that all your thoughts come from yourself?

Have you ever paused to wonder if your feelings, preferences, likes and dislikes truly belong to you?

Did it happen to you that maybe they came from outside, from other nations, and you unintentionally embraced them as your own?

After reading all the above words, do you still accept that you control your mind or that the forces beyond you regulate it?

If you do not screen the thoughts that invade your mind, you will stop being a free person and encourage every thought to rule your life.

You can object and say that the thoughts that go through your mind are yours, but are they?

Have you consciously and attentively generated every thought that came into your mind?

As we have said before, we are exposed to immense knowledge every day, coming from relatives, friends, teachers, podcasts, TV, newspapers, and social media, of course.

This information is a reflection of our opinions and emotions.

Why do outside forces affect your mind and your life?

Why let other people's thoughts dominate your mind and life?

Do you want to be able to choose your feelings, or do you want to enslave your views and thoughts to others?

If you leave your mind open to any thought that passes by, you put your life in the hands of others, and without knowing it, you will acknowledge their thoughts and behave in accordance with them.

Every person is influenced differently by external surroundings. Many thoughts and suggestions that we neglect, and those that motivate us to take decisive action. Thoughts about things we enjoy have more control over us than other thoughts. However, if we are constantly subjected to thoughts and ideas that we don't care for, we will inevitably allow them to influence us.

Everyone has the interests, aspirations and dreams that he or she might have fostered since childhood. It is likely, however, that some are the thoughts of parents, teachers, and friends who have remained in their minds.

How To Take Charge Of Your Thoughts

Have you ever felt in your mind that you did not like something? It may have been rude, sinful, cruel, or frightening. You may even have wondered, where did that come from?

Your mind is the most important weapon you have for creating good in your life, but it can also be the most destructive weapon in your life if it is not used correctly. To regulate your thoughts to affect the way, you live your life.

More, precisely your subconscious influences your perception and thus your understanding of reality.

Life is straightforward, you are what your thoughts are, you build on them, and when your thoughts come out in words and deeds, you get them back with outstanding accuracy and that is you! Your thoughts and words will transform your World; it is the use of our speech and actions that is the cause of our fears and stress. We have justified in our mind; the external circumstances in our World explain our disorders and anxieties, which is a FALSE belief.

Manipulate your mind as a powerful workman's tool when finished, switch off the tool and put it down to rest, until the next time your powerful instrument needs to be used again. Compel it to learn new skills and talents. Apply and progress in your life, so you become the expert, with a degree of discipline, and an open mind and willing to use your sense as a powerful mechanism, allow it serve you in your life.

We make a program in our mind which is implemented the way we desire, but we are not happy with the results; if you don't develop a great program, how can you predict excellent work! Then you might ask me what was missing?

If you give a cup of milk to a child and warn him, "be cautious not to spill the milk," there are more chances he will spill it, don't you think so? Yes? Is that a mistake made by the child? My response is no.

Why? Because a malicious program (your caution) was developed, instead of "keep the milk safe," you could do a lot of work, you are wondering what the difference is well, the first statement was a pessimistic one that demonstrates that you don't trust the child. It also suggests that he might drop it. He does spill the milk, a negative mindset always gives an adverse outcome; in the second statement that you make, that child thinks on his own to make a self-decision. It shows your trust, so a positive idea will do the job because you've programmed it positively by saying what's going on.

The example demonstrates an essential part of how our subconscious mind picks up such tiny signals and makes us do what is intended.

So many of us are victims of our minds. Our thoughts are always turning; few of us know what each day holds: Tired, we use our regular upper caffeine. Overworked, we are going to put ourselves down with substances that drain and cause blockers—unable to stop the computer at night, we turn to sleeping aids.

This is the best that our culture expects us to do; however, we can do more.

The truth is, you can take control of your mind and your emotions. It's not that easy. It is tough.

It has taken me years of regular practice, and I am still far from extraordinary. However, having gone wider than is "fair" (e.g.., hours a day of training), I've found enough of the map that I can see the rest of the area.

Step 1: Start With The Thoughts You Want To Think About

Imagine that you are in a dark room, fumbling around the wall for a light switch. Do you stop to think about how you came to be in this dark room? Are you contemplating the mechanism that led you to walk into a dark room without a flashlight or knowing exactly where the light switch is?

No, you can find the light switch and illuminate the room.

Too many of us want to get right to the "fixing." We want to break down the mental mechanisms that hold us under tension or up at night.

We are going to sleep more comfortably if we stop worrying about it and concentrate on the things we like.

Ask yourself, how do I want to think about it right now? Do I want to be stressed, irritated, or at ease? Do I want to think about this or that, or feel like it is under control?

In Possession of Your Mind, what thoughts do you have? Are they good thoughts or bad ones? If bad thoughts appear, crush them as quickly as possible and try to be aware and catch yourself before a dramatic story has cooked up in your intellect, replace the dialogue with your list of positive intentions, affirm good, and do not allow the mind to cook up a whole lot of drama and garbage. As that's what is to happen, lending rise to more fears and anxiety.

The mind movie happens to all of us, from personal experience and been in enough situations to know when the triggers happen recognizing them and knowledge on how to train yourself, altering your story to a positive one, thank God you became aware and caught them in time.

Ask yourself, if I was in that state of mind, what kind of thoughts would I have? How does it feel to think about that? Before embarking on any decision big or small, ask, will this be right for my greatest good or does this feel right in my heart, will it benefit me or others.

Only playing a role in your mind, you're going to get a "reality transition."

Your brain knows how to do this, and like clicking a button, your brain is going where you're going.

When you decide, at the moment, to concentrate on something good, you use your mind (attention) to direct the mechanism that we call the brain.

Step 2: Describe The Behaviors Of Who You Want To Be

Step 2 is challenging, it's not going to get through initially. It's no small feat to gather the courage to say to your subconscious, "No, this is how I'm going to behave and think right now."

Doing this exercise day-in and day-out, is positively tricky.

This is why the monks spend their lives away from all worldly "agitations" and associate themselves with people and an atmosphere that is only favorable to shaping that way of being.

Few of us are trying to cut off the rest of the planet to train our minds.

But you too, can build on behaviors and rituals that will make it simpler and more stable for you to manage your thoughts eventually.

You've pictured the way you want to think in the previous step. Now, imagine the person who has been thinking this way for a lifetime. If you are trying to banish fear and anxiety, imagine a version of you that feels confident most of the time.

If you are trying to become a more compassionate person, imagine an edition of you that's unshakeable and always at ease.

Are you in charge of your mind?

What does your day look like?

When you wake up, how do you react to the grogginess and urge to hit the snooze button? Do you give yourself time? have you got your morning rituals to set you up for a winning day ahead? Do you smile when your eyes open? Are you grateful for a few moments? Do you appreciate the day ahead? That you are alive and consciously make yourself think and feel cheerful in the morning and for the rest of the day ahead?

If you are stuck in traffic, how will you respond to the delay in your day?

What if you are drawn into a confrontation or conflict at home or work? How do you feel and respond? Are you proactive or reactive?

After the day is over, how are you going to disconnect?

Imagine yourself going through a full day as this person, and record how you respond to outside stimuli. You're never going to have complete control of your day's external stimuli, but you do control how you respond.

By doing this exercise, you're offering a map to your brain, showing it exactly how you want your mind to be. I am going to respond this way, when I am faced with a loved one in a state of suffering or an angry client. If I am under an oppressive deadline, I am going to think that way.

These everyday habits are not small at all. Much like 20 pushups a day is going to strengthen your body, which is mental muscle conditioning.

Step 3: Get Into Your Burning Passion

None of this is easy to do. A famous bit of drugstore psychology is the saying, "The toughest part is getting started," but that's crap. The most challenging thing is to remain committed to the course to gain the momentum.

Go to any gym on the 3rd of January. I can guarantee that it will be flooded with people who "get started" with their resolve to get in shape this year. Go back to the same gym into the first week of February, and most of them will be gone.

Anyone could get started. There are a lot of people who registered companies but never made efforts to expand them. Also, some people quit their jobs to start new lives and ended up in the same place.

What is uncommon in the world is the people who have stayed the course, who have endured the frustration and struggle that success requires and have changed their lives for the better.

Winners are not all famous, but they all have one thing in common: Intense Passion.

Do you have a burning desire to control your mind?

The Dalai Lama, probably the most professional human being on the planet to "monitor" his mind, mediates 3-5 hours a day. Severe! And people do manage to meditate straight through for 2-5 hours in any one sitting, they are extraordinary human beings!

If you want to master this subject, you need to tap into passionate desires and decide what you're willing to do to manage better the way you think and feel.

At least, integrate these three steps into your Daily Exercises:

Each morning, take 10 minutes to ground yourself. Breathe deeply and slowy, concentrating on your body's sensations. Allow yourself to be centered in the moment. Think back to a time when you knew exactly what you wanted, and now welcome that feeling.

Kill negative self-talk all day. I was talking about this in my anxiety post. Our internal dialogue is also a source of anxiety. Much like you would turn off a TV show that irritated you, know that self-doubt is just a discussion within your mind you might end up with.

Until you finish your day, rehearse the performance. Michael Phelps calls it "Putting on a video tape." He took time every night before bed to picture himself swimming and winning the gold medal. At night, imagine how you want to think and feel to have the most fantastic day.

Step 4: Develop A Psychological Toolbox.

A Mercedes needs different components, equipment, and skills to work than a Porsche. The same is true for each one of us.

The nuances about what motivates and challenges you will be different from what motivates and challenges me. On a day-to-day basis, you can come across circumstances that continuously test your mental self-control.

And you're going to have to find the resources that work for you to resolve these obstacles.

For example, there are two places that I have been dealing with for some time because of my hostile mind. The first one was my lack of ability to shake off a depressive situation. If something went awry early in my day, it was difficult for me to feel optimistic or act motivated for the rest of the day.

To smash this, I have created a technique called "Prevention is the Cure" a four-step procedure that helps you to improve your neurology no matter what's going on around you:

1. Force a smile. The feeling of your muscles responding to a smile — even a fake one — signifies to your brain that it is time to be happy.

2. Thrust your arms out in the open. Any quick burst of movement will relieve stress, get your blood flow and circulation pumping, that will get you back in the moment.

3. Always make use of encouraging words, anything precise as "Yes! I did it" or "I'm going to make it" You will work wonders by overriding "your negative self-talk" encouraging you to be vocal, close to primary screaming.

4. Exhaling deeply allows you to let go of all the stress and relax. Please put the book down if you will and do it right now, take some deep breaths and let it go, multiple times.

Get Rid Of Anxiety By Taking Charge Of Your Thoughts

You can eliminate anxiety by getting the right positive attitude. Anxiety could lead to insomnia and, in combination with stress, can cause high blood pressure and a host of autoimmune diseases as the immune system is weakened. Exercise your mind's strength, gain ownership of it, and don't allow it to adhere to fear and anxiety.

You can get rid of anxiety by taking the following steps:

Start Looking At How Fear Enters

The sensation of dread is generated when you see a picture in your mind that you do not accomplish your ideal situations or a loved one is in a bad state. We project these images in our mind's eye, which means that we can also take charge of our leaders, instead, cast a favorable impression. You can witness yourself attaining your goals.

See that your loved ones are well, happy, comfortable and safe, I say these affirmations everyday for myself, for the ones I love and all of humanity, I wish or send them out in the form of a prayer, I tell myself 1st. "May I be happy, may I be well, may I be comfortable and at peace" Then, I picture someone I love very much, and I say, "May you be happy, may you be well, may you be comfortable and at peace" And lastly, I bring everyone into the picture, even those that I may not know or be in contact with, "May we all be happy, may we all be well, may we all be comfortable and at peace," and "May all the suffering end in the World." Maria my qigong teacher always ends the meditations in her Yin yoga classes with similar affirmations and prayers, these blessings do wonderful things.

Prayer Is One Of The Best Ways To Overcome Feelings Of Anxiety

Anxiety arises when our desire to succeed clashes with our mental image of failure. Prayer generates a bond of confidence and comfort in a most Merciful God and produces a calm and peaceful serene feeling that flows into the body. The surface is that nothing can go wrong because Heaven is on our side, and that God, the most potent force in existence, is protecting us.

Deliberately Transfer Bad Feelings Out Of Your Head

Refuse to concentrate on bad feelings, and keep the focus on the optimistic thoughts.

Think About A Previous Case In Which You Have Had Tremendous Success

Please take a moment to appreciate the feeling of success and translate it into the present. Feel the confidence in every fiber of your being. Feel assured that you are still in a position to accomplish the challenge at the moment.

Take Note Of How You're Talking About Yourself

We all talk to ourselves every day. Your self-talk has significant roles to play in erasing the anxieties. If you keep reminding yourself that unpleasant things will happen, you ramp up your stress level, that will make you feel more nervous. Your subconscious mind acknowledges the information that has been reinforced and then what do you feel? Your emotion goes into a state of panic. Deliberately utter positive words to yourself, and it will keep you calm, centered, healthy, happy, and confident.

Meditation For Mind Control

Meditation for mind control is about taking full control of our life and reasoning. Think about it, around sixty thousand thoughts and ideas pop into our heads every day. Many of these ideas are not our own and originated from the relentless flooding of media ads, newspapers, the internet, other people, etc. I am sure you agree that most of these thoughts are not safe and desperate to handle.

The fact that our minds are continually being bombarded with unnecessary garbage and waste of our precious time is a severe concern for us. Why? -Because our emotions are driving our lives.

If our thoughts decide our lives, then we can alter our situations first by changing our mindset. How are we going to do that? Yes, it's going to take time, and work, but the good news is that it is quite simple.

Views of the thoughts you have about your Life

The first step is to give a check-up to our thinking life. We need to take time to concentrate on what we are thinking.

Take note and review your thoughts over the next few days.

Consider the following:

- Thinking about yourself (ability, personality, fitness, etc.)
- Thinking about others (God, spirituality, families, etc.)
- Thought about your life purpose, career, present and future.
- Thought about any other aspects of your life.

When you review and analyze your feelings, consider which ones are safe, constructive, efficient, and advantageous to your life. Ask yourself if they're going to help you step in a better direction? Then determine whether you're going to let them stay or give them the boot.

For example, you could think of becoming a financial disaster and continually failing with everything you do. Your mind will replay past failure events and come up with many explanations of why you are sure to fail in the future, so you end up living in deprivation.

What do these kinds of negative thoughts do? It takes away all the hope of being financially successful and seeking happiness, and on top of that, it makes you think you should settle for less or accept poverty.

By realizing that this kind of negativity is just detrimental, you can then try to avoid it, by balancing it with ideas that would be beneficial and effective in your life.

Mind Control For Right Thinking & Right Living

After you've offered your thinking life, a check-up and decided the thoughts are no longer allowed to exist in your mind, the next process is to take responsibility and make some mind control clean-up.

To eradicate negative, detrimental, unwanted thoughts, instead constructive, motivating, and beneficial ideas must be substituted. We can't just tell an unwelcome opinion to stop and go away. We need to replace it with the right thinking.

For example, you tell those opinions of debts or insecurity to stop, and you take charge of your mind by substituting those negative thought patterns with a successful thought. God's word is full of hope for success. He requires us to be blessed to be a blessing to others. We are encouraged to meditate on the thoughts that will lead us to a successful life and salvation in our hereafter. But God is not just going to step into our minds and clean up our ideas for us, this world exists on cause-and-effect methodology. It is something we have got to do, with his comfort and support.

It is said we have dialogue with God through our prayer, and through meditation, God is in dialogue with us, so I highly encourage us all to pray and have a meditation habit in our everyday existence. I know it is not easy initially, from experience but doable if we schedule our prayer and our meditation practice for 5-10 minutes into a routine preferable at the same time every day consistently just like our daily shower, brushing our teeth or eating is a habit and part of our daily rituals.

Take Responsibility For Your Thoughts

Bear in mind: your thoughts result in your emotional wellbeing, and these affect your life. Then why aren't you in charge and taking care of them?

Refuse to allow your mind to concentrate on the thoughts of negative past experiences, current difficult challenges, or any other debilitating thoughts that fill your mind with complaints and disappointment. Refuse to keep your life geared towards continual torture.

Bottom line: please read a fantastic book, As a man thinketh so he is, by James Allen. Decide which thoughts you want to hold, and then substitute negative thoughts with constructive ones that will lead to results. Meditate on the teachings of the Scriptures of God's Word and take care of your life's view with Grace.

CHAPTER 3
BELIEVE AND RECEIVE

"Believe in your infinite potential; your only limitations are those you set upon yourself."

Perhaps there is something you desire in your life? Is that a new career, a home, a spouse? Or would you like to earn more money, or is the New Year's Debt Free in the plan? Okay, what if I told you that you can have what you are searching for using three words? Ask Believe, and Receive. These three words are powerful.

Some individuals do well to use these three words and can get what they're looking for or become more generous. Nevertheless, some people have a tough time implementing this in their lives. In this section of this book, we're going to reveal precisely what to do to apply it to your life and achieve what you ask for, but always note that TIMING plays a massive part in receiving what you have requested.

Do you believe that you can maximize excellence? Is your answer a no? Then you might need to change how you look at things, so the things you look at, can start changing.

Believe, and you're going to get. when I feel out of balance or a negative thought triggers me off, I affirm, ***"I am safe, secure and I trust"*** that immediately has a positive affect on me, I say it over and over, until I feel the emotions are incongruent with the affirmation, also this is the same declaration to rehearse for balancing your root chakra.

These terms have been presented many times, by many, in many ways, but they all amount to the same thing. Most people are in the same place, looking at things the same way they've been for years and they wonder why things don't change.

For them:

They have not lost the weight they expect to lose, or they will never be satisfied until they attain all their goals in life. They are searching for the Perfect Company etc.

Thinking they know how to Master Good, but they do not. Still, devoting considerable time to things that are futile that don't matter more than preparation and execution. Some people have not done what they set out to do because they don't believe they can have or are deserving.

Let's be straightforward.

If you realize that you will have whatever you desire or be what you want, you can, and the funny part is that it comes quite easily.

If you're not satisfied with where you are at right now and want to make your life a lot better, you have to decide to change. You've got to change the way you think about what you want and who you want to be.

You're probably going to have to do some stuff you've never done before. Norman Vincent Peale said: "change your mind and change your universe."

Will, you arrange some time for yourself to concentrate both personally and professionally on your life? If you haven't started yet, set aside time for yourself and spend some time with yourself. For you will obtain what, you believe.

Have you ever thought of having a very viable business or profitable career and being financially independent so you can have more free time?

How does that make you feel? Do you feel comfortable when you think about those things? Do you feel secure, happy, and generous when success brings you more freedom? when I believe I can, I feel that way too.

Do you know you've got all the answers inside of you? The real challenge is to dig through all those feelings, all those months, years of indoctrination, and reform the way you reason. Start believing that you're going to get what your thoughts are all about. Okay, I mean, honestly believe it.

Or, if you like, you could sit around and start believing that you cannot possess the things you desire.

And witness as all the good things in LIFE eludes you.

It will require you to do some stuff you never accomplished before. Yet, inside of you, you can be whatever you want.

Ask, Believe, Receive – The Formula For Making Things Happen

Does it seem relatively easy? All I must do is inquire, then believe I'm going to receive it! The hardest part of the three for most is not ready to receive.

The reality is, most of us do not request, many are too busy concentrating on believing for quite a long time, and even very few are genuinely ready to receive. Ask, Believe, and Receive is a method that has been shown to function numerous times again.

Many of the achievements begin with a challenge; there is a question that makes room for possibility. I always say to my children, "You don't ask, you don't get." Asking can take multiple shapes. It might be a written list of priorities or a prayer that you say every day. It might be a wish you were dreaming about every night before you retire to sleep.

But whatever you ask, whether you make it possible by simply writing, reasoning it, or speaking it aloud, you make it a genuine possibility. If you propose a wish, a dream, a goal out into the world, the world goes to work on that appeal. Your mind is going to focus on it.

Too many of us are scared to ask; maybe by asking, you're afraid you're going to be disappointed. Perhaps you want something you don't think you can have. Your passion can be so intense that you can't talk. But to obtain it, you must inquire first. By writing, wondering, or asking about it, you're setting the wheels in motion. This is the beginning of the journey to get to the desired effects.

What are you searching for? What you seek is also in search of you. You may have a health problem that you want to heal, or it could be a relationship or friendship that needs rekindling. It could be a business target. Whatever it is, it is time for you to get serious and write it all down, wish it or script it. The first step in answering, "Believe it and, receive it," is answering.

If you keep a journal, please write your questions. If you are a thinker, you want it to be in your mind. If you are going to say something about your wishes, declare it out loud. But every day, you have to keep asking for what you want. The intention of visioning your request is to plant the seed into your subconscious mind in the present here and now. Your mind is going to focus on your questions while you relax and do other stuff. Many opportunities will come your way to orchestrate the request closer to actualization, and sometimes you will not know- how or why.

Believing you are going to excel is the second most potent weapon you have with you right now. It's available 24/7. No one can take it away from you. When you believe you're going to win, great things happen. If you feel you're going to heal you will. If you feel you're going to get a raise, you will. If you believe you are going to find your soul mate or friend, you will.

When you claim your inquiries are constructive, as if they have already occurred, you are expanding your mind to the power of a happy feeling. It's a simple concept that's been around for years.

When you trigger that force, you begin to align your universe with your queries. Incredible things begin to pop up in your path to drive you towards your goals. You're going to get the things you've asked for.

You're able to receive it now. Often I go back to my journals and see a question or a target that I've overlooked, and it is already happened, I received even better than I had imagined.

Here's how to inquire, believe & receive the Law of Attraction at Work.

1. The Mindset Of Daily Gratitude: when you are grateful you can't be anxious or angry simultaneously, Tony Robbins taught me many things, and my favorite is a morning ritual, a wonderful start to your day, a few minutes of moving and breathing, gratitude, prayer, for healing, solving, strengthening, celebrating your wins and service to the creation, then lastly you visualize and set your goals for the short term and long term, and how you will attract the right people and circumstances in your life to make it all a reality.

Below is a list of a few of my favorite gratitude affirmations, that you can add to your journal or make up your list. Say these declarations or incantations out loud everyday with belief and emotion, witness the miraculous changes that happen, they will make you feel instanously wonderful and grateful for the blessing and the precious gift of life.

- Thank you; I love you.
- Thank you for the fresh air.
- Thank you for my beautiful heart, lungs, and organs.
- Thank you for my beautiful life.
- Thank you; I am safe secure, and I trust.
- Thank you for the delicious food and drinks.
- Thank you for work, exercise, rest, prayers, and meditation.
- Thank you for my spouse, children, and family.
- Thank you for all my blessings.

Make a long list of everything you are thankful for the simple and the profound things in your life, things that you have and the things that you would like to attract in your life. You need to be very precise and have a very nice extensive list, that will make you feel so happy and thankful! Things you're grateful for every day, the smallest things matter as much as anything else. Let this be your crucial mindset. Nothing interacts better with the Law of Attraction than the Attitude of Appreciation. Gratitude is a potent force of energy and power. This is an important point, and you should write it down; gratitude is a joint force of energy and power! Simply put, you're going to get back what you are giving out, and you will feel good inside.

2. Emotional Intelligence: it's about keeping the feelings controlled and free of any ego. Ego is the significant divergence from the energy field that we call the Law of Attraction. When your emotional intelligence is active, you will find that you are much more forgiving towards others, a better listener and that you seem to have an infinite supply towards compassion and kindness. How is your EI or emotional intelligence score on a scale of 1 to 10?

3. Clarity & Concentration: When you make time to remove all the regular noise or distractions, it's pretty easy to concentrate on Asking, Believing, and the hidden weapon of the three, the genuine desire to Receive. Much of the time, we're never able to receive. ***"Oh no, I couldn't have allowed that"*** Have you ever heard yourself say that? When things are offered or given, accept them as a gift, as life is such a precious gift, so flow freely with the attitude of gratitude.

Receiving completes the energy exchange, no matter what the object is. The more frequently you receive, the more your receiving channel is available. When things come your way, they come with energy; then always receive it freely and happily. Things are going to come to you more quickly since you don't have any obstacles. The world wishes to send you stuff every day, so be aware and ready to accept. It may appear odd, but your desire to receive is just as critical as your desire to give.

4. Multitasking: Caution, GUYS! This refers to so many things that we're trying to do in a day. Anyone who is in an extreme multi-tasking phase is doing a great disservice to themselves. No time to be thankful, no time to be calm or get centered, with consistent feelings, and least of all, any focus or concentration. Multi-tasking by default refers to keep fitting things in. It's pretty much zero standards. Requesting, Believing, and Obtaining is a way of thought, one that needs some attention to detail, so set aside some time to do it properly.

If you rehearse the Ask, Believe, Receive process, you will see the results. Asking is the same thing as setting a goal and praying. To believe is to have the confidence that you will excel with certainty. Receiving is a reward for asking and believing. What are you asking for?

How To Follow & Activate These Basic Steps Of ASK, BELIEVE AND RECEIVE

Step 1: Ask For What You Want

The role of asking for what you desire allows you to be specific about what you long for. Ask, Believe, Receive, does not work unless you are absolutely sure. It would help if you are confident in your mind to get a direct signal from the cosmos. If you are not sure, you're going to send out mixed alerts. If the world picks up conflicting frequencies, you're going to draw mixed effects. Being explicit and direct about your needs sends out specific and direct signals to the world, and this makes it possible to reach your goals.

For example, if you say, "I want a better life," the world does not have anything to do with it. A better life could mean winning the lottery, but it could also mean, you want a home, a spouse, children, or something work-related so be extremely specific about your requests.

If you request what you would like to be unique, such as "I want a job that I love to do, which allows me to use my creative skills," the world will join forces to bring that employment.

When you inquire about something, you present a definitive choice. You've placed your request with the human world, and you trust you've been heard. Think of the act of asking for orders from a menu or directory.

Asking is always about wishing something specific. Sometimes asking is simply a matter of finding a response. When you have to make a hard choice and don't know what to believe or what to do, you ask. Know, the Rule of Attraction asks, "Believe, accept, give back what you put out."

For example, if you decide on which one of your friends is to be your maid of honor, you may say, "I wish there were a simple way to decide who to choose." The universe will orchestrate an event to give you the reply. It could come in the form as a text message that gives you some insight. Or maybe one of your mates will unexpectedly become unavailable.

The only thing you've got to do is inquire. Rest assured the world is going to fill in the rest with impulses for you, with which you will receive your answer, and now you must act.

Step 2: Understand Your Thoughts Have Strength

You have to trust, what you wished for will be yours. In secret, Inquire, Believe and Receive is all necessary, but to believe means understanding the power of your thoughts. The moment you asked, acknowledge, and realize your answer is coming. What you desire already resides in the unknown, and the world has begun to form alliances to introduce it to the manifest. Have full trust in yourself. The world is a mirror reflecting your prevailing feelings, so assuming that, you already have what you wished to remember when you receive it.

If you believe that you will receive what you asked for, you must relax, be patient, and wait for it to show up with effortless ease.

The trick is not to dwell on not getting it yet. If you are staying on the fact that you don't have it, you're going to rely on the memory of not getting it. The strength at which the thoughts emit is not getting it. Note, The Hidden Inquire, Belief, Receive is a three-step process. So, the only images you are sending back are without what you want.

If what you asked for does not happen right away, don't fear that the world hasn't heard or understood you. Trust that the world has understood you and that what you want is already awaiting you in your future.

For example, if you buy tickets for a cruise around the world that doesn't leave for four months, you will still feel confident that you'll be on that ship in four months.

Feel the sense of security with the law of Attraction. If you were sure, there could be no doubt about your future.

HOW is not your concern? How you're going to get what you want, what you're going to need to do, and how it is going to be brought to you, is left for God to give the universe the order to deal with.

Many of us have never encouraged ourselves to do what we do because we can't see how we're going to get it.

Let the world take care of the way it does. All you need to do is ask and trust that you will receive.

If you're having trouble believing that you're going to get what you are hoping for, claim to believe. Once upon a time we were children, we made ourselves delighted with excitement. We declared and believed we were explorers or superheroes. We envisioned our inner warriors are protecting and guiding us. We were free to let our minds go wild with whatever fantasy we liked. As adults, our rationality and logistics are always getting in the way. In the Law of Attraction, of Ask, Believe, and Receive, the frequency we are emitting is our guidance system.

Making you believe as an adult will make you believe what you have wished for is already yours.

For instance, if you want a new Porsche, make sure you drive the Porsche down a winding road. Daydreaming of yourself sitting inside the car and visualize everything you can about the interior, the smell of the new leather seats, the dashboard the more visual you are the better, you are behind the wheel driving this beautiful sports car. Please do this before the imagination starts to feel like it is a reality.

I can tell this works, and has happened to me, what I was visualising for my life became a reality for me, when I reflect back, everything has manifested into the manifest because I had already asked by daydreaming.

I recall, I was bored staring out of the school classroom window, I was dreaming about a sports car and a different life to the one I was living, I guess unconsciously I had realised, I was not happy about certain things in my life at that tender young age, and dreamed of better, I had no idea that material objects would manifest, we do not realise the power of our minds, what they can dream up, these incredible thoughts, intentions, visions and goals.

I was 12 years old, I believed, and made the decision, I had already received. I think it really helped me to daydream, to have something else to look forward to then the dread to have to live through traumas of early childhood.

The observer of self-limiting beliefs, arguments, resentment, drama, and not being understood. Witness to the constant battle between the adults and not allowed to express feelings. We survived ongoing conflict and negativity. At that immature age, we absorb it all without any judgment or understanding and get affected by it all later in life, and we end up mirroring those same patterns in our adult lives.

By dreaming of achieving better, living a wonderful life, these feelings gave rise to an inner knowing and happiness. I had forgotten about the outcomes and like any child got on with life, going fast forward. I am in my early 20's, living a beautiful life of my dreams. I had a home and independent life. So, this is a clear demonstration, of how we can manifest whatever we desire. Being in a state of happiness, whatever the circumstances are externally and internally, always reminding ourselves of being cheerful, grateful, and thankful for everything we receive and wish to receive.

I have also experienced the opposite, for when we are ungrateful, for all the abundant gifts, blessings, unconsciously the very things we love, also get snatched away, so be very mindful about the opposite being very true!

If you can see what you have asked for, you're going to start believing that you've already received it.

Step 3: Receive What You Asked For

This is the last step in The Hidden Ask, Believe, Receive. Even before you have received, the act of feeling that you have received communicates powerfully with the universe. Feel all the sensations that come with receiving what you asked for. You feel happy when you get what you want. Why would you like something which does not make you smile? You wouldn't do that. Ask, assume you have received it, and be very grateful to receive it.

When you are happy to receive what you want, you're sending out your receipts strength. The intensity of receiving is the frequency with which all great things are brought to you. Get on this intensity, and get exactly what you requested.

Conceptually, it might seem clear cut. But when you try to apply it, you will encounter the full swing of contradictory thoughts and emotions, moving mainly around the issues of fear, guilt, shame, doubt, and the question of "Am I worthy?" Don't worry – you are not alone, and these contradictory emotions are just certainly part of your insight, confidence, and instinct.

Let me share with you a story by Katherine Hepburn to illustrate the secret through which you can receive more of what you desire.

Once when I was a teenager, my father and I were standing in line to buy tickets for the circus.

Finally, there was only one other family between us and the ticket counter. This family made a big impression on me.

There were eight children, all probably under the age of 12. The way they were dressed, you could tell they did not have a lot of money, but their clothes were neat and clean.

The children were well-behaved, all of them standing in line, two-by-two behind their parents, holding hands. They were excitedly chattering about the clowns, animals, and all the acts they would see that night. By their excitement, you could sense they had never been to the circus before. It would be a highlight of their lives.

The father and mother were at the head of the pack, standing proud as could be. The mother was holding her husband's hand, looking up at him as if to say, "You're my knight in shining armor." He was smiling and enjoying seeing his family happy.

The ticket lady asked the man how many tickets he wanted? He proudly responded, "I'd like to buy eight children's tickets and two adult tickets, so I can take my family to the circus." The ticket lady stated the price.

The man's wife let go of his hand, her head dropped, the man's lip began to quiver. Then he leaned a little closer and asked, "How much did you say?" The ticket lady again stated the price.

The man did not have enough money. How was he supposed to turn around and tell his eight kids that he did not have enough money to take them to the circus?

Seeing what was going on, my dad reached into his pocket, pulled out a $20 bill, and then dropped it on the ground. (We were not wealthy in any sense of the word!) My father bent down, picked up the $20 bill, tapped the man on the shoulder, and said, "Excuse me, sir, this fell out of your pocket."

The father understood what was going on. He wasn't begging for a handout but certainly appreciated the help in a desperate, heartbreaking, and embarrassing situation.

He looked straight into my dad's eyes, he took my dad's hand in both of his, squeezed tightly onto the $20 bill, and with his lip quivering and a tear streaming down his cheek, he replied, "Thank you, thank you, sir. This means a lot to me and my family."

My father and I went back to our car and drove home. The $20 that my dad gave away is what we would buy our tickets.

Although we did not get to see the circus that night, we both felt a joy inside us that was far greater than seeing the circus could ever provide.

That day I learned the value to Give.

The Giver would be greater than the Receiver if you want to be considerable in expansion, learn to Give.

Only if you Give, can you Receive more. The Givers heart becomes the Ocean, in tune with the Almighty - The Source.

Love has nothing to do with what you expect to get - only with what you are hoping to give - which is everything.

In conclusion, if you use this mechanism, trust and believe, that what you want in life will happen, it will happen. However, note that timing plays a part and do not give up on what you believe.

CHAPTER 4
WHAT SELF-BELIEF CAN DO FOR YOU

"Great things happen to those who are persistent, believing their dream is here now, being humble and grateful."

When it comes to achieving success, nothing is more critical and persuasive than belief in oneself and self-confidence. If we want to be successful, self-confidence is more essential than intellect, ability, history, or anything else. Also, people who have self-confidence and believe in themselves are healthier, happier, better connected, inspired, resilient, and behave in a balanced way, when things do not go as forcasted.

In life, we often find ourselves in circumstances where we are affected by others. It's an inevitable part of life. As children, we want to fit in, be accepted and appropriate, satisfy others, and earn recognition and respect. It's a vital part of life. If we fit in, we can stay as part of the crowd or tribe, be looked after and stay safe. If we are rejected, then we may find ourselves ostracized or cast out and lose our validation.

Fitting in with the crowd makes us have a sense of belonging, taken care of, and makes us feel safe. If we are ignored, we may find ourselves marginalized or expelled.

Self-belief must be nurtured as part of our creation. It is our degree of trust. Children from stable, caring families also find that they have self esteem, feel worthy and confident when they take a gamble on trying out something different and new. They are motivated, and even if they struggle to produce the best performance, they will find that they are appreciated and rewarded for their bravery and commitment. They have faith in trusting themselves and their abilities and they gain self-confidence.

So what does it mean to believe in yourself and to have self-confidence? Broadly defined, it is a feeling of trust in our judgment, capacity, and quality. It's often known as self-efficacy. This, influences almost every part of our lives, including how we think, feel, and act. That's why it is so critical.

We have all made mistakes, witnessed loss, and felt discontent in our lives and we will all be tested in life. I know I had more than my fair share of trials, tribulations and relationship disappointments, you just can't please everyone, I wonder sometimes to myself, when will the drama end. Some of us have even been exposed to betrayal, suffering, oppression, and even had our hearts broken.

All these encounters affect a person's self-confidence and trust in their choices, decisions and abilities in this life and we give our power away just so we must fit around other people's drama. Luckily, there are ways to build self-esteem and confidence even if it takes some effort and time. It's worth noting that our past does not have to determine our future. The only thing of importance is the way we behave in the present moment now and focus our attention on the high frequency vibrational energy to gain confidence and momentum, and leave what does not serve us or engage with or give away our power over to others.

So let's look at how much strength we have when we trust in ourselves.

The Power Of Self-Belief

Large numbers of people every day, enable others to create doubts about their potential to achieve their goals, make them feel vulnerable and inadequate, and generally lead to the low quality of their state of mind, and therefore, sometimes to the quality of their lives in general.

Self-belief is nothing other than faith in who you are, what you believe, and how you feel. It does not mean you're always right about these mentalities, as long as you believe them and behave accordingly, they will affect your emotions, attitudes, and life.

Self-confidence is such a valuable quality to have, as, without the willingness to believe in your value and deeds, you will fail to achieve your maximum potential and live a less successful life. If you don't believe in your potential, you're not going to meet the expectations you are capable of. If you do not believe in your own decisions, you will become clueless and less likely to take risks. If you don't feel secure in your own body, it can affect your contentment and trust.

It is well known that self-confidence can lead to mental well-being. Often those who lack confidence are more likely to feel inadequate, socially insecure, nervous, embarrassed, paranoid and doubtful. This is heightened in day-to-day life by the presence of social media, as we, are continually overwhelmed with unrealistic expectations of body image and lifestyle; this may make people paradoxical about their own lives as they compare their lives to celebrities.

As far as self-belief is concerned, comparisons could be detrimental, as they can bring your faith even more to a shallow level, making you feel like you're never going to be good enough.

Without self-confidence, we will never set out on the road to achieving our goals, and we need to believe that we have the potential to get there – by believing in our ambitions, we can have a vital purpose in our lives. I've always been told, "If you believe, you will succeed."

While this might seem insignificant, I firmly believe that if you go into something with an optimistic mind of "I can do it" attitude, rather than "I don't think I can do this," you are more likely to do better. In part, I disagree with the widely used expression, "If you don't believe in yourself, no one else will." Self-belief encourages motivation and self-confidence, which will make it easier for others to want to give you opportunities in life. This is not always the case, however! For example, I may not believe in my intellect, but my parents or my partner does, and they help me, boost my self-confidence.

When self-confidence is grounded in integrity, honesty, intelligence, and reverence for your higher self, it will drive you toward your hopes, ambitions, and aspirations. When self-confidence is valued in all respects, it will move you into a future that will be real for you one day. Essentially, your dreams are just as real, as is your trust in them. So, if your ambitions are not yet a reality-think-that, maybe your self-confidence needs serious tasks from the inside out.

When you allow perceptions and external influences to affect your self-confidence, you will always come up short of your aspirations and desires. Please, get this if you want the future you are dreaming of becoming a reality for yourself- Start concentrating on growth, progress, and trust in who you are, who you become, and who you are capable of being. Is it a straightforward task? Not at all. But I want to keep on encouraging and reminding you the effort, time, and commitment you make are worth it.

Spiritual Confidence & How You Can Acquire It

Spiritual faith derives from your belief, your relation to the Divine Presence. This may be the occurrence of a spiritual awakening, or it may be because of increasing faith in the way you allow the Divine presence to communicate with you.

This kind of confidence appears to be attributed to an intense spiritual awakening. The foundation of faith is belief and of acquiring knowledge. Focusing on belief is a crucial acknowledgement of the eternal Spiritual reality.

Genuine Spiritual Confidence

Genuine spiritual confidence is when you live the wisdom guidance, and the Divine lives in you as expected. Otherwise, it's all about your acquisitions and Performance.

There is only one way to be outstanding, and that's to learn to obey the acknowledgement of your soul. Your soul knows how to understand the universe in you more than you can interpret.

You can think about everything you want, but then it's a lack of concentration. You are living from desire. Spiritual trust is the assurance that what you desire will be granted to you because you follow the Divine Will. That's the only thing you need to reflect on and learn to express through you.

Genuine spiritual faith and the spiritual Law of Attraction come from practicing the question, "How may I serve?" This is the central challenge of living as an accomplished human being. This is the issue in the theory that is fundamental to the Western mind. Everything is transaction motivated.

The goal of the spiritual intention in developing spiritual faith is not about you, but about you willing to follow the Message as it is to be expressed through you. Spiritual faith is where you know how to fulfill God's purpose, which joyfully becomes the core focus of your life.

You must put this intention to your intellect and try to make it apparent. You learn to be complete so that you can become a source of accomplishment. The less there is about you and your dictation to the world, the more quickly it comes running towards you effortlessly, when you stop running after the world, leave the glitter and illusions, the world begins to come running towards you.

How To Build Spiritual Confidence

Allow me to start by reminding you that the confidence, I am encouraging is the understanding of spiritual awareness. This is an extraordinary way of being in the world. This is where your concentration is not on obtaining what you want, but on letting your inner guidance communicate through you.

Because of this Core Purpose of being open to the Divine Will, "Everything is extraordinary to you." You will be an important addition to the common good of all, which is also your greatest virtue.

This is going to happen through you. You are certain this will happen for you, but you're not going to try and control the result in some way that you determine. Your pleasure will be in the confidence that comes from being the servant of God.

Here are some significant components to establish true spiritual faith.

- The Intention.
- The Silence.

- The Trust.
- The Ascension.

These combined effects will give you the groundwork to understand how to become spiritually confident.

If you make this your routine spiritual exercise, you will succeed in the true definition of that word. It's going to make you correspond with your intellect.

So, let us discuss these four pillars of building up our spiritual faith.

Intention Is Greater Than The Action

Nothing occurs without the force of intent. It is the force that drives production. This is a spiritual method to build up spiritual confidence, so the purpose must be one that aligns you with the communication with the Divine.

If there is no communion involvement with the supernatural as a direct and personal experience, then there will be no encounter of spiritual faith. It is from this feeling of relation that such trust is built up. This is an invitation to true unshakeable spiritual faith - One that does not rely on visualization and overthinking.

Spiritual confidence is your belief and your spiritual knowledge and closeness to the supernatural. This knowledge is the result of a clear understanding that comes to Grace. You cannot build up spiritual confidence without the explicit knowledge of the Divine intention as it passes through you.

The Power Of Silence

Spiritual confidence grows in proportion to the extent to which you enjoy solitude and stillness. This stillness enables you to think about and imagine what you want. This is what you're doing, not living by just existing.

Every spiritual person knows and loves the paradoxical forces of peace and silence.

Nothing is happening in the beginning. This is where most people stop the process of designing and building up their spiritual confidence. They're not sticking with the exercises. Nothing is being done, and it seems somewhat illogical.

That's exactly what's going on, but you've got to stay in silence to know the magic that's going to pour through you.

The term "confidence" is translated as "having faith in." This is true faith. That is the confidence not knowing, but ready to be learned. It is not a blind faith.

The Power Of Trust

The word confidence is a less controversial word than faith. In this one word, the entire spiritual process of awakening may rightly be summed up. This is the ability to trust the Still Small Voice inside and the strength of the Inner Wisdom.

This is where you learn to believe that you are a part of the Divine Root, but never separate from it. Trust in the way the Divine will work through you is the pillar of unshakeable faith.

Trust requires you to step into the uncertain about making it possible to know the supernatural intention. This is different from deciding what you want and then committing to envisioning and affirming it.

Spiritual Ascension

Spiritual confidence is an embodied faith. I have seen much too much spiritual disembodiment promoted by the numerous teachings misinterpreted by the Western psyche in my spiritual quest.

One such teaching is the teaching of detachment. A lot of spiritual confidence seekers have taken this to mean separation from emotions. Typically, this is a feeling they're still disconnected from. As a result, they become much more disconnected and etheric.

You cannot experience spiritual faith by ignoring feelings of rage and remorse. These are the facets of your personality you need to incorporate. As the writer, Colin Tipping said.

– Radical Forgiveness – advises, "The only way to heal is to feel it."

How To Gain Self-Confidence & Believing In Yourself

List your past successes and accomplishments.

Many of us are unfairly harsh on ourselves. We prefer to remember our errors and weaknesses than our successes. Yes, we have all fallen short and we've blundered as anyone has at many points in life. Yet we have also managed to effectively tackle tough challenges and achieve the things we should be proud of. Rather than what we have done, we prefer to reflect on our failures.

Create a list of all the things you've accomplished in your life, big and small. You will be surprised how much you've accomplished that you are forgetting and give yourself accolades. Even more important, add achievements to your list every day, and read it often. You are more competent than you can ever know.

Focus Your Attention On The Solutions & Not The Problems

Whenever we are short of self-confidence, we prefer to concentrate on the negative things rather than positive ones. Instead of trying to produce ideas, we get daunted and distracted by problems. Whenever you are overwhelmed by your fear of taking on a challenge, strive to find ways to conquer future obstacles instead of worrying about something that could go wrong.

Avoid Negative People

Just as we must associate ourselves with optimistic and happy people who boost our self-confidence, we should eliminate those who do the reverse. Please, stay away from toxic friends and people who thrive on futility and might cause you to regret later on asking yourself, "why did I waste precious time" at least reduce spending time with those you know who will suck your energy, respectfully excuse that company. Suffering, complaining, gossiping, backbiting, harming, blaming, playing the victim and mischief making, loves the company of people, so do your best to avoid at all levels to save your soul!

List Your Strengths

As we mentioned, most people are faster at talking about their defeats than their achievements. In the same vein, we still prefer to concentrate on our shortcomings rather than our abilities. Often, we have to depend on the closest people to figure out our qualities because we are oblivious. Create a list of your strengths (ask your family and friends if you need to) and paste it where you can see it every day. I assure you that you've got a lot more power than you remember. You've got self worth and talent that you often ignore.

Groom Yourself

Have you ever felt much better after a haircut or a warm bath or dressing up with your best clothes. The use of essential oils for a massage or manicure and pedicure. Your mind, body, and soul will thank you for the much-needed "TLC." Appropriate grooming helps us feel happier, lighter and better about ourselves and enhances our trust within.

CHAPTER 5
ABUNDANCE MINDSET VS. SCARCITY MINDSET

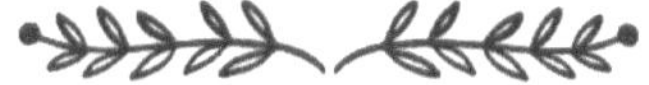

"Once your mindset changes, everything on the outside will change along with it."

We all like to fantasize about becoming financially successful. It remains a fantasy for most people, and nothing more. Why is it?

It's because most people don't think they're going to achieve that goal. They may not be pleased in their present situation, but they are comfortable –being in their comfort zone is one of the greatest enemies of SELF development.

Many people believe that the wealthy have secrets of abundance that will never be revealed with the world's commoners. The fact is, the wealthy have secrets. But they're not exactly what you expect. A simple shift of your mindset will pave the way to satisfying as abundant as you want to live.

Examples of abundant mentality vs. scarcity mentality are as follows. When you change your perspective of the achievement of prosperity, it will become clear how true the dream exists. Mindset transformation is the single most significant factor that influences our failure or success in everything we try. Why? That one's mind is the outward manifestation of expectations, fears, dreams and beliefs about a specific subject. We're thinking about particular problems, i.e., parenting, achievement, well-being, etc. a collection of values that we've stored up.

We also have an overall attitude that contributes to our perspective on life. As far as the former is concerned, if a subject such as parenting is discussed, We enter the "box" where all our beliefs are kept and we respond based on our feelings about the issue. For example, one might assume that parenting is challenging, stressful, tiresome, and not worth the trouble. Whenever this subject is brought up to such a person, they may say, "I don't want children-they're a lot of work!" because their parenting is connected to a lot of negative feelings and perceptions. They don't have a particularly good parenting mentality.

The views, as mentioned earlier, are founded on the experiences that people have. The subconscious mind is healthy and operates solely because we do not know where we store these values based on our own experiences. One individual can find that he or she has a balanced diet, exercises, and generally keeps balanced and easy to stay healthy and happy. Their experience with keeping up with good health is optimistic, and they have optimistic values in the box called "health." It is not a problem for them, which is something they do with comfort. On the other hand, another individual could panic if a health issue is imposed because they are constantly dieting and are unable to shed weight or remain healthy. This person is unlikely to have something positive to say about the matter and will likely never be productive in achieving good health.

The other aspect of the way of thinking that arises relates to one's overall perspective on life. Again, this is centered on experience, but a larger scale. Depending on how people get on in various areas of their lives, values, expectations, fears, and desires are placed in a box called "me." Because of these convictions, one becomes either an optimist or a pessimist.

These two facets of the mind (the confidence in certain subjects and the overall view of life) go hand in hand when achieving success in any area of life. As described above, most people take for granted that we are continually contributing to the beliefs that influence our minds.

That's why it's crucial to be conscious of the individuals, societies, and values that "expose" us. Developing the winner's overall thinking takes a lot of effort. The subconscious mind ultimately influences everything we are and do, it is a powerful machine that consumes almost everything.

To be successful, in anything be it mental, physical, emotional, psychological, or spiritual, one needs to focus on cultivating a successful way of thinking that sees one taking responsibility and accountability for who they are and what they are doing.

Having a victim mentality has nothing to do with one's pursuit of excellence. Dedicate to improving yourself, remain driven and empowered so that you, too, can grow the winner's mindset and become whatever and whoever you desire to become.

Changing Your Mindset

How are we going to change our thinking? We will quickly shift our thinking by repeating to ourselves that we're ready for success and the necessary adjustments to make it happen. Every day we will realize that success is what we strive for, and we deserve it. We are going to think positively of ourselves and the collective difference we will make with our contribution to the world.

With consistent thinking in progress, we will slowly lower all the shackles that keep us in the old way of thinking, because it has been our habit to think negatively. Still, with patient repetition of thoughts, we will have a new method of thinking about ourselves as someone worthy and deserving of a good life and greatness, and any occurrence that does not help support positive thinking we will turn away from it and continue to live the successful best version of the way we want to become.

We will write down in detail all the good things we have, and when we make mistakes, be motivated and encouraged to do better afterward, because success is promised to us. We're going to blink at any loss and let it pass us by without being too angry because we know it's coming with the thoughts we've talked about before.

We now have the chance that what we think today will bring us success in the future. We would be glad to work on ourselves and our mind since we know that this is the only way forward of changing our minds, behaviors, and actions when something shocks us. The behavior emerges naturally from the condition we found ourselves.

Mindset Shift

The mindset shift concept is a persistent mind that has become normal for us to shift from the way we think.

This condition is created by a constant thought that has become normal and natural for us to think about. We think of the state in which we are, and slowly, construct a positive or pessimistic or a fixed state of mind.

Success needs the growth mindset because it allows us to think positively for ourselves, quickly overcome the challenges ahead of us, and look out to win for opportunities we have to change our lives for the better.

We can change our mindset with wisdom, within ourselves on the path to change what we like, and convincing ourselves when we revert to the old way of thinking about our past that causes us to respond in a turbulent manner.

To change our mind, we need to want to be a different person than we are at any given moment. It takes a lot of dedication and willpower because we will have to work hard and guide our thinking to what we want to experience.

How To Change The Mindset

We're going to direct our attention to that we want to say about ourselves, MINDSET SHIFT IS SUBSTANTIAL, if we're going to think of ourselves as successful, if we don't do well at work, we have to disregard reality and convince ourselves that we are successful, competent, that everything around us, is happening for our greatest good, that all is well, that while we don't see improvements instantly, they will surely come, that we bring within ourselves the success and all the requisite characteristics.

We have enough patience, focusing on oneself and one's emotions are the most difficult mental work that one can do because it involves being immediately aware and keeping a watchful eye on what we think at all times.

When we begin to think negatively and when we start to fear failure, which will always happen, we must instantly guide our attention to the intended goal in which we are already succeeding. We will create a successful version of us, because of our perseverance, we will resolve all the challenges that will lead us to the intended result.

How To Change Your Mindset To Be Positive

Changing our way of thinking to a constructive one would persistently steer our thoughts to what we want to do in our life and a constructive vision for the future. We will bring forth about ourselves the best version of ourselves, and calm down when unwanted things happen to us. We will repeat statements that validate what we want to become and that this is a natural series of events for us to bring us to heightened awareness.

We will emphasize that we deserve a healthy, beautiful, and fulfilling life, that we will accomplish everything. We prefer by establishing high performance standards on ourselves, with persistent improvement on our thoughts and proficiency, as this will appeal to us through a new outlook towards ourselves and the activities around us. We will learn new habits, new skills, enthusiastic to master new reactions to events and people around us that will lead us to a better position for positive results that we want to achieve inherently.

How To Change Your Mindset For Success

We are going to change our way of thinking about success by continuing to think of ourselves as a successful individual who deserves a good life and will encourage us to earn a successful income.

We are going to reiterate and use transformational vocabulary which compliments our success and it is now a part of us and we will do whatever it takes. We are going to put ourselves in the mood of our greatest version and ask ourselves, what thoughts we need to think to feel good now? We will concentrate on our success-oriented mindset and replace any negative thinking that impedes us on our road to good thoughts about ourselves and the work we have to do.

To be effective in our minds, we must start thinking differently about ourselves. We must see every mistake as an experience and a blessing that will educate us on a new attitude that we would not have encountered. Don't be so skeptical about yourself anymore, for any critique you make goes back to an old way of thinking that does not lead to a good life, but a struggle to stay in the comfort zone and that will make you think you have a comfortable life and not allow you to progress further, or accept life and become complacent and go back to the same old patterns. We must eliminate the old habits and on to the new best version of ourselves and who are these role models, we are going to seek out to help us, get to our desired destination.

We need to be at the forefront of our awareness, as we think about our future, and through diligence, we will achieve a new way of thinking that will offer us well-being and increase the trust that we need to take measures towards our intended goal.

Through this method, we will allay any fears that we are always in the habit of thinking and turning to those thoughts that help us switch to a better future. From the perspective of a successful individual or a successful version of us, we think who is successful and who undoubtedly thinks positively of herself and recognizes that she has already accomplished the objective that is now our vision.

Some Differences Between People With Abundance Mindset & Scarcity Mindset

If you choose to view the world as scarce, you become therefore fearful of what you can lose. Or you can view the world as abundant and full of opportunity.

Scarcity mindset people:

1. Are always fearful of losing things or running out of resources and money.
2. Focus on the short-term of every choice.
3. Evaluate decisions based primarily on risk and loss.
4. Create sadness and jealousy in their lives.

Believe there's just one pie, and anyone who gets a big piece of that pie is taking it from someone else.

Scarcity mindset people are somewhat difficult to help. It's too much work trying to convince them that they can be successful in anything they set their mind or endeavors towards.

They don't believe they can do a job and love, which earns them a salary they deserve and follow their passions for prosperity or the market isn't too saturated for them to succeed. Truth is they just don't believe in themselves and this limits them in achieving their goals.

Abundance mindset people however:

1. Always believe the world is full of opportunities for them to explore.
2. Focus on the long-term of choices.
3. Evaluate decisions based on gain and development.

4. Create happiness and success for themselves and the people around them.
5. Believe there's no limit to what's possible and what they can achieve.

3 Important Mindset Shifts For Spiritual Growth

Our way of thinking forms our reality. Either they can help us grow spiritually, or they can leave us trapped. I am a great believer in continually exploring my mind and how it affects my life and my spiritual development.

In this part of the book, I share with you what I believe are the three most critical changes of mindset that will support you on your spiritual quest. I hope they will be as beneficial to you as they have been for me.

See Your Past With Gratitude

Coming to terms with your past is one of the most important things you can do for yourself. I've seen amazing things happen in a matter of minutes when people choose to look at their history with love and appreciation.

All that has happened in your life has taken you to your present level of knowledge and built the life you are now living. It has led you to want a deeper connection with yourself and the world. Your experience has transformed you into someone who's searching for a high-vibration life. Otherwise, you would not be here reading this, and you would not be involved in mind shifts for your spiritual self or self development. If your past were different, you'd read something else, somewhere else, while focusing on something entirely different.

In some of the most challenging times of your life, you have molded yourself and built the perspectives, characteristics, skills, and the mindset, you have today. Every experience has encouraged the growth needed to get you to the beautiful soul that you are today.

The more you can accept and respect your experience, the easier it becomes to communicate with yourself, your inner world, and your source of energy. Start with forgiveness and move towards gratitude.

See Everything As Assisting You In Your Spiritual Growth

You have an option to view your life in whatever dimension you want. When you choose to see things that are happening to improve you rather than damage you, your journey will be a lot more exciting and rewarding. It will also increase your confidence in self development, because you lift your intensity and connect yourself with the higher reality by making this change.

When something terrible or challenging happens in your life, ask yourself:

1. How's this going to help me?
2. What did I do to attract this and what do I have to learn from this situation?
3. What is fractured inside of me that will help me to heal?
4. What is it that gives me the ability to release or let go of?
5. How do I see it from my highest perspective?

Focus Internally, Instead Of Externally

You've got all the answers you are searching for inside of yourself. All you need to do is to know how to find them. We live in a culture that teaches us to explore beyond ourselves. A culture where we are encouraged to appreciate the external and the way things look and neglect the internal and the things we can't see. So, it is not shocking if you're searching internally to feel odd or unusual at first.

You might also have been doubtful about getting all the answers inside of you. When I began my journey, I just wanted to find a master who could give me all the solutions. What I found instead was a great teacher who showed me how to communicate with myself and my inner guide.

My many teachers taught me the value of doing my daily prayers, my yoga practice based on the tradition of holistic Hatha Yoga and the eight limbs. They taught me the importance of regular meditation, practicing pranayama, living in harmony, forgiveness, non-violence (especially within myself), connecting my body-mind and soul through (physical yoga postures), and the importance of self-enquiry-study.

CHAPTER 6
FINDING YOUR PURPOSE THROUGH SPIRITUALITY

"It's not enough to have lived. We should be determined to live for something."

You may have always wondered about your purpose in this life, I guess you do that a lot? It could have bothered you repeatedly. Is that right? Do you find the answers to all your concerns? All these questions also trouble our nerves and take a lot of time to fade away in our minds. Don't get confused, relax, and take a look at your life, with a view that is completely different than ever before. It will make you understand what you've been missing so far! I'm sure that, this question will pop up in everyone's mind and soul one day! Have you ever thought about why this issue comes up? Let me enlighten you! Every person has come to this planet with a destined intent, and now and then, their "inner voice" reminds them of it, and that's why this question keeps ringing in our heads frequently.

It would help if you found the answer to this question of your soul and inner knowledge of how to live your life's purpose and be happy. How do you go about that? There are two groups of people in this world-The first type are the ones who are not concerned about the reasons behind their presence in the world, and who continue to live a careless and chaotic life without much effort to find the meaning of life, and those who are responsive enough to come up with frequent brainstorming thoughts to get their actual purpose in life. People with a future vision turn around their fate and at the same time, wave the whole atmosphere around them to put things right in an attempt to help, the people around them find their life meaningful, the experience of which they were not aware of up to presently.

Importance Of Having Meaning, Purpose & Spirituality In Life

You must have a mission in life to feel contentment with your life. Famous examples of life purpose may be to excel in the right profession, contribute to your society, raise a family, grow creative talent, achieve an educational objective, support others with their challenges, resolve addictions, or issues of unhealthy childhood. When you know what brings purpose and meaning to your life, you are more likely to go beyond your personal needs and positively affect others. When you start to realize your real intent and ability, you begin to step far above your individual needs and make a significant impact. This, on the other hand, gives you pleasure and relieves your stress and anxiety. Besides, it gives a sense of clarity, and you work hard to expand others as an inner motivation.

Let me share with you the story of a man of how his purpose and good deed kept him alive.

There was a Jewish man named Joseph, who had a bread kitchen, a town, in Crown Heights, Germany. He frequently said, "Do you know why I am alive today?"

He said, "I was a child, at the time when the Nazis were killing the Jews mercilessly in Germany."

We were on the train being taken to Auschwitz by the Nazis. Night came, and it was creepy and cold in that compartment.

The Germans left us on the tracks throughout the night, and for quite a long time, with no food. There were no covers to keep us warm. The snow was falling all over; cold breezes were hitting our cheeks each second. There were many people on that horrible cold night. No food. No water. No asylum. No covers.

The blood in our bodies began freezing. It was turning out to be ice.

Next to me, there was a darling old Jewish man from my old neighborhood. He was shuddering from head to toe and looked awful. So I folded my arms over him to warm him up.

I hugged him firmly to give him some warmth. I scoured his arms, his legs, his face, his neck. I implored him to attempt to stay awake and alive.

I energized him the entire night, I kept this man warm along these lines.

I was drained and cold myself. My fingers were numb, but I didn't give up scouring heat into the older man's body.

A long time passed by. Finally, morning came, and the sun started to sparkle. I glanced around to see the others.

Regrettably, all I saw was solidified bodies. Everything I could hear was ghastly quiet. No one else in that lodge was alive. That freezing night murdered them all.

They passed on from the cold. Just two people survived: the old man and I.

The old man survived because I kept him warm that frosty night and I survived because I was kept warm by serving him.

May I disclose to you the key to endurance in this world? When you will warm other hearts, you will stay warm yourself. When you uphold, empower, and motivate others, you will also find support, consolation, and motivation in your own life.

The key to a joyful life, when we regard others, we regard the self, when we satisfy people, they will fulfill us.

Bear each other's weight and satisfy the commands of God.

How are we going to discover our life's purpose? To get an answer, you have to ask yourself, Am I satisfied with the education I have received? Do I have a special gift that I can share or any artistic talents? Have I built up my faith? What do I want to do with my life? What is my passion for life? Is there something that I would love to accomplish but have not been able to acquire yet? What improvements do I need to make to be able to realize these principles in my life? Is there someone I respect and admire, yet I haven't been able make a connection? What skills do I need to be able to understand these statements? Do I have unique gifts that I have not entirely recognized in my life? What challenges will I need to commit to excel to my maximum potential?

Spirituality

Just as having significance and life purpose is important because it helps you relieve pain and anxiety, spirituality also helps over come your worries and fears. Spirituality requires the understanding and acceptance of the Highest Power over and above your intellect and your will. When you build a relationship with your Creator the Higher Power, you will be inspired; you will have the peace of mind and the implicit encouragement you will obtain from your Higher Power.

Whenever you feel uneasy, you should have recourse to your relationship with your Higher Power and ask for strength, guidance, and truth to the straight path and encouragement to help you deal with your worries and issues. It's an experience that requires perception and relationship with something that transcends yourself.

For our reason, we refer to the Almighty power of GOD which may be abstract or very straightforward. Nature, flora and fauna, scenic views, and the magic surrounding you are all part of the secret discoveries. They are all expressions of the Higher Power's existence. THE WHOLE WORLD IS A MIRROR OF GOD and all his creations are expressions of his greatness.

With spirituality, you build self-confidence that will finally help you cope with the struggles of life. You are not depressed in the face of a problem, but self-confidence allows you to stay persistent and enable you to achieve your goals. Moreover, if you believe in the Greater power of GOD, it gives you an awareness of unconditional love. This is a kind of love that is preferable to romantic love.

Unconditional love allows you to show compassion and love for others without being judged by others. As your bond with the Highest power deepens; you begin to feel a greater degree of unconditional love, which starts to manifest in your increased ability to give love to others and to experience more of it coming in your life. Your worries have been reduced, and you will enjoy life more. You often support others by encouraging them and making their sense of unconditional love more straightforward.

Developing a relationship with your Creator can provide support for decision-making and problem-solving. When you interact with the Source, you will rely upon His more excellent knowledge to help you solve your problems. Often it's beneficial to imagine GOD as if you see him all the time and he is your guidance. First, of all, you need to calm your mind by doing progressive muscle relaxation. Are you hurting from severe anxiety or pain? "Don't worry everything will be okay" everything in this world is temporary, the situation, the issues, or something else that worries you will pass.

I have a conversation with GOD as if I see him all the time, or I know He is watching me all the time, and that helps calm all my insecurities, anxieties, and fears, whenever I feel helpless or in any difficult circumstance. Trust me; I have been in many, then I know I must hand over my troubles to him, you can do the same; this is the state we must all cultivate.

Think about this for a few moments before you have it clearly in your mind. Confirm over and over with as much certainty as you can, "I hand it over to God he has all the knowledge in the seen and unseen." "I surrender this issue over to you, my Almighty Powerful Merciful Creator, please God help me solve this issue." Repeat this phrase quietly and gently and with emotions. If you're visually inclined, imagine that you are going to find your answers—this aims to create trust and confidence in your Higher Power.

An attitude of modesty and surrender is the key to this part of the process. Often it is helpful to imagine a bright yellow or white lights of mercy raining over to the spot in your body you feel nervous or concerned about. The solar plexus, known as your stomach center, is typically the part of the body where your anxious feelings reside. When you imagine this light entering the parts of your body, it helps break down your anxiety. You may want to extend this practice for 30 to 45 minutes to feel the bond to your Creator. When your anxiety or worry comes up, do the exercise again until you have perfected the process of breaking down your fears.

You can strengthen your bond with your Creator, to access the spiritual vibrational energy that is pure and holy. Through daily prayers, reading of divine revelations, holy scriptures, inspirational literature, meditation practice, and the use of spiritual affirmations. They appear to re-affirm your faith, to give you self-confidence and courage to face the challenges of life.

In this way, we can see that faith can help inspire and give you the confidence to follow through with your recovery program—we all face difficulties in life-related to jobs, relationships, schooling, and personal circumstances. If we don't have these struggles, we are not going to evolve and learn. By overcoming the adversities of life, we become stronger and better prepared to cope with stress. Yet we need the tools to be able to meet the challenges of our lives.

What matters most is how you cope with the depression at a time of adversity. You have two options either to split up or face the challenge with a sense of adventure, delight, bravery and excitement. Becoming depressed and nervous will not fix the problem. If you feel frustrated, trapped, and confused, you can have a recourse to your spiritual faith, practice the Higher power visualization and have the conversation with GOD and discover the meaning and intent of your life. You can see that life will look more beautiful and that your mindset and view of life's problems will alter.

You will fill the inner vacuum created when you did not have any purpose and meaning to your life. People engage in volunteering, support the needy, educate children, provide community programs for the mentally ill, join the Rotary Club, support the Red Cross, find happiness in life and reach some satisfaction. Anyone can live a life for themself but living for others and doing community service requires bravery, dedication, and a capacity to rise above oneself to have maximum potential. This kind of satisfaction would result in the greatest happiness and lack of concern and anxiety in life. It also helps keep you entirely up to date as our great leaders, e.g Mahatma Gandhi, Abraham Lincoln, Mother Teresa, and several other distinguished luminaries. As you become self-realized, your self-esteem will increase, and you will be in a better position to deal with your problems.

Finding Your Spiritual Purpose

Life has a lot of objectives. Many of them are accomplished in your daily activities, and you do not think of them as objectives. Yet you could say that meaning and purpose are motivated by every choice, every experience, and every role you have played that teaches you lessons about yourself, your interactions, people, organizations, and life issues. The training and development that has or is occurring from each experience moves you towards heightened understanding and can be seen as a goal in your life. Some of you may want to look wider and see the central theme or spiritual purpose for your existence. Knowing your spiritual objective is a motivating and exciting force in one's life. Are you confident of your spiritual purpose, or already thinking of another assignment?

Life's purpose summons some people in a specific, transparent manner and others in one particular or unspecific way. Some people are very conscious of their goals, while others are not. Some people actively pursue their spiritual purpose, and others allow life to guide them not to give them much thought. Confident people do not need to describe what they do as a spiritual objective, and others do so. If you have approached mid-life, it is customary to pursue a more profound meaning and intent for your life beyond your family or work's involvement. Some of you may feel the desire to make a valuable contribution to humanity, to support society and the world by using the knowledge garnered from your life, to become more self-realized.

Some of us may not know our spiritual-self, mind, and God has chosen us to share our life to a particular path. Without describing it as a spiritual goal, you may have had a great deal of inner desire to achieve individual goals or build and use specific skills and abilities many times as an art form. If you were to turn around and take a look at your life, you could see some significant trends that point in the path of seeing your goal. You may have had a deep desire to create or refinish furniture, grow orchids, know the names of local trees and birds, write editorials in your local paper, or start your own company.

The ability to cultivate and appreciate one's interests and skills can be seen as recognizing a spiritual meaning. If it is to the benefit of others, that is great, but the fact is, if it adds more joy, happiness, and compassion to your life, and benefits to the world.

How do you get more in-depth to find a spiritual sense and intention that will inspire, enhance, and enrich your life at any age? Let's take a look at two methods. There is a yin, gentle, passive, or flowing approach that enables your spiritual purpose to find you. There is the yang, the directive, the involved, or the quest for an answer to seeking your spiritual meaning. Many of you have had a mixture of both systems.

Now take a look at your own life. If you're not yet certain of your spiritual intent, do you want to examine your awareness to find out? Perhaps you have a vision of accomplishment, a wish to take another step towards finding your spiritual objective? Do you have complete knowledge of yourself? Have you gone through inner healing? Have you asked yourself about your purpose in life and also your actual contribution to the world?

"How do I align with the divine guidance to navigate my life?" These and many more questions will come up when you are ready. Those of you just starting on a spiritual journey note that it's not a sprint, and we don't measure ourselves based on someone else's life. We open when our timing is right. Many people discover their meaning in existence when they are in the process of self-discovery and inner healing. Others don't realize that consciously for a long time.

Many of you on the yang side of the equation can use the Life-Purpose Resources to help you initiate a more in-depth phase. Get your journal out so that you have a record of your responses and observations for further research. Ignore any negative self-talk that tries to destroy your spiritual bloom. Dread and uncertainty may attempt to stop the inner directions getting to you by telling you that you are not competent, advanced enough, or deserving enough to function in life more extensively.

Know that it is your divine nature that you want to tap into that is beyond any negative influence. Enable the process to occur as you bind the masterpiece of your greater purpose together. Honor the right timing for you. Pay close attention to your dreams, write down your insights, thoughts, wishes, visions, ideas, hunches, or feelings you get during your journey. Some people interpret their news in a quiet voice that communicates to them, others see images, and others have a feeling or impulses for answers.

After you've taken the Life-Purpose Inventory, mediate your responses, and write in your journal every day until you feel a sense of guidance or understanding.

You might feel the role you're going to play and the area you're going to play in a big picture of life, or you might just see the next step or two for you. Write down all your thoughts; they are significant even if they seem to be insignificant or boring. Take it seriously, for example, if you feel the urge to get home, to organize your things like drawers, files or anything that needs to be put in order. By decluttering or removing what, you do not need, you are opening the door to allow what you need to come to you.

Suppose you have the impression of simplifying your busy lifestyle. In that case, it will benefit you to re-examine your activities and give priority to your immediate needs and principles to build a strong base for your spiritual journey which is just around the corner.

You may feel you need to go on a specific diet, identify and treat one of your addictive behaviors, or start a fitness routine. If you complete these worldly steps, you will be given the next step. The trick is to follow each step and to realize that you are progressing along your spiritual journey. Continue to conquer uncertainty and negative self-talk and keep going. Someday, you will turn around and observe where you were two, five, or ten years ago, and you'll be happily shocked that, by taking one step at a time, you have come so far.

Honor your reluctance and the moments when you feel no desire to bring forth into motion what you know you need to do. Listen, and you will find that you need some nurturing or finishing some loose ends in your life, maybe repairing one of your relationships, quitting a career, or changing your negative thinking. You are not going back when you're going through a time of need for help.

Remember that it is just as precious a spiritual aim as is to raise a child, to nurture a farm, to support your family and friends when they need love and help, to cultivate one of your gifts, to get to know one another, or to find a solution to a problem, as it is to be the leader of your club, an artist, a mother, a pro athlete, or to teach a class, or write a book. The main thing is to be your true self and to understand your spiritual purpose(s).

If you take one step at a time or get the big picture when you explore your spiritual meaning. Only go with what works for you. Your inner self understands you and how to teach and inspire you. Thank goodness you don't have to be in control, so indulge in the process of finding your spiritual intent.

Some people have a particular call, and others have a more general intent. You have a unique function that only you can serve, otherwise, you will not be here, or you will be appointed. Do not underestimate the importance of every one and your mission. The greater whole of humanity wants your special note in the symphony of creation.

CHAPTER 7
PRACTISING MEDITATION
FOR HAPPINESS

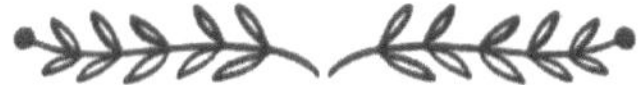

"To understand the immeasurable, the mind
must be tranquil & still."

What comes to your mind when you think about happiness? Is it a feeling you are seeking but never quite achieving, or a state of mind that you can tap into if you have the proper knowledge? What do we all have in common here? What is driving us? What is it that both of us are searching for? We are all seeking to escape discomfort, struggle, and frustration. We want to be relaxed and happy and to feel a sense of well-being in our lives. Yet, most of us are in the wrong places searching for happiness.

Happiness is a mental state — a raw feeling of contentment, satisfaction, and joy in life.

In this contemporary age, people get too distracted with a lot of things. And with all these worries, it is hard for many people to experience inner happiness and satisfaction.

If we asked ourselves what we were looking for day after day, the answer is straightforward happiness. Everyone's goal in life is to be happy, and this expresses itself in many ways. To others, buying material things makes them happy. Others find comfort in food.

With all the anger, frustrations, fearmongering, insecurities of loss, conflict, anxiety, and suffering in the world today, it can be challenging to find joy in life, but that's where meditation on happiness can help.

And we all have witnessed much pain, chaos, confusion, misery, and struggles; it is not surprising some of us feel like the external world does not have any dimension of happiness to offer.

You might be asking yourself, "How can we be happy when others act up towards us?"

If you want to achieve your destiny and become the absolute best version of yourself, you must take the time to nurture the joy within. Meditation informs us, the pleasure is inside of us.

We can all be content if we look inward. As simple as it sounds, too many of us find this idea daunting. Here lies the question: How do we find happiness in meditation?

Relying On External Situations Results In Dissatisfaction

We are actively seeking pleasurable circumstances that we believe can bring long-term happiness. We are attracted to money, strength, prosperity, assets, friendships, safety, and the like because we think they can give us steady satisfaction. But most of these pursuits do not contribute to the desired result.

We are seeking happiness in the wrong location because we cannot see things unchangeable in existence.

Every circumstance, everything we might benefit from to ensure this happiness will happen. External objects are not able to give us lasting satisfaction.

There is always a limit on what external things will get us. When curiosity and excitement end or circumstances shift (as they always do), our minds turn to various degrees of frustration, which is articulated as a means of agitation. We strive to get relief from this upheaval by reaching out for answers. Deep down, we are disturbed, and we do not see how we get stuck — we are like a fish that is attracted to the bait. This cycle can be called the "reset discontent mode."

Of course, this does not mean that we should be cynical about our lives and our universe. The world offers many delightful, pleasurable things, such as positive relationships, meaningful jobs, healthy living, and stable circumstances that provide comfort for a certain amount of time. But the problem is that they are not wholly accurate. Situations are shifting. Friendships are coming and going, a family member passes on, our children are growing up and leaving home, our budgets are changing, and our health becomes less stable.

We need to be more practical. No one wants to encounter traumatic circumstances, such as physical discomfort, emotional discomfort, or death, but they still happen. We cannot control many things about the outside world, but we can control how we react to them. Most of the frustration we feel is due to our inner state of being, not only external circumstances. This is where meditation comes in.

Mindfulness Meditation For Success – The Science Of Happiness

Meditation and genuine happiness can be a way of life—Success-meditation is best for your comfort and lifestyle.

You can see the theory of happiness often in your daily life.

I mean, being more fulfilled and happier than you have already been is an exceedingly challenging task to perform, but not in the process until you get the hang of it and get to know what you have learned exactly. I am always saying that you are going to excel in everything you have set out to do in life with prayer and meditation for your well-being.

The path you have chosen that has led you to your present situation has not been a couple of days or months in the making, but it has been a long and stressful path spanned over several years. It took you as long as you were alive to end up being what you are and who you are today.

It has taken you too long to do just what you have done and to get to your present condition.

Does Meditation For Joy & Happiness Work?

Putting in the effort to exercise and believe in mindfulness and happiness and meditation for success, and what you possess in your life is what you need.

If you are delighted with how your life is going, congratulations-do more of what you have done, and you will get more of what you have already had in your life.

If your present conditions are less than what you want, or you are far from precisely what you desire, you might want to consider mindfulness and happiness.

Meditating on joy and happiness will help you and some simple changes you will have to make in your life.

Failure to make those improvements will make you discover that you are looking for the essential things that you want in your life as the years go forward.

Is Happiness Created Within?

If you have read any of this, that can seem a little dull when it comes to meditation on joy and happiness and might not sink in at first, causing ridiculous reflection on performance.

As the Miracle Course teaches, "Don't be scared to try going deeper," because when we get to the heart of who we are, it can be genuinely thrilling.

I want to say that before you take lightly, rather than profoundly, how mindfulness and happiness meditation can help you in your life, ask yourself if you want it to be real-then for your gain, and please allow yourself to see it as real.

In this day and time, with all the essential things we must handle in our lives, it is tough to remain on the right level and be happy all the time.

Meditation Gives Us Access To Our Happiness & Well-Being

The mind retains the inherent qualities of well-being and clarity that lie underneath the superficial level of frustration. The main aim of meditation is to access, identify, and improve the mind's optimistic nature. The more we can do this, the less we need to acquire external circumstances for happiness. The more we can focus on our natural, optimistic aspects: affection, contentment, healthy-living, and happiness.

Accessing our innate happiness and inner well-being is one of the most significant accomplishments. They are always with us, and they do not rely on anything outside. Nobody can take them away. They rely only on us and affect everything in a positive light. It is like uncovering a secret treasure inside. To get access to this treasure, we start by focusing on the inside – and for this, we need training.

Meditation is this kind of preparation. When we meditate more, we gain trust in our fundamental, inherent goodness and sound health; this unlocks our potential and gives life a significant purpose. In this context, the question "Does meditation make you happy?" answers itself. Meditation does not make you happy – it activates the "happy" that has always been there.

How To Meditate & Increase Happiness

Okay, so here is a quick but amazingly effective gratitude meditation that you can do every day to improve your overall happiness.

Take A Moment To Relax Your Mind

Sit or lie down for a moment and take a few long deep breaths and exhalations, concentrating your mind on your breathing. Breathe in slowly, breathe out slowly and thoroughly.

And when you breathe, you cultivate non-attachment to your emotions. As soon as you find yourself worrying about anything other than living, remove the thinking gradually.

Think of your feelings as train cars going through the station. You are on the platform, watching them go by. But you do not get to ride them and let them take you somewhere else.

You are simply observing them as they go by and letting them move on without you and then gently returning your attention to your breath.

Be Grateful For What You Are Experiencing

If your mind starts to settle down, I would like you to give thanks for all that you are feeling at this moment – first, beginning inward with your most recent encounters and working your way out.

Thank Your Mind & Body

Give thanks to your subconscious, which helps you to think about all your thoughts. Be thankful for your eyes, which allow you to see the beauty of the world. Express gratitude to your ears that let you hear the world's beautiful sounds, and then to your mouth that lets you taste the world's deliciousness in all its various forms. You are thanking the Creator for all your blessings in your life.

Be thankful for your arms, your hands, and everything that they allow you to do — such as holding a baby, reaching out to toss or catch a ball, or a falling child. Authoring a book, typing a study, driving a car, playing an instrument, creating a piece of art, cooking a meal, hugging a loved one, or making love.

Thank your heart for pumping blood through your veins, arteries, and your lungs, allowing you to breathe, and for your throat and tongue to let you speak and express yourself. And be thankful for your legs and feet, for making it possible for you to walk, run, leap, and dance.

Be Grateful For Your Present Environment

Be thankful for the chair you are sitting on and for the people who put their time and effort into making that chair—the money that helped you buy that chair, or for the person who gave it to you.

Be thankful for the coffee cup next to you, and the delicious coffee you had is now running through your veins, making you feel more awake and alert.

Be thankful for the clothes you wear, the person that made those clothes, and the work that gave you the money you needed to purchase them.

Thank Your Extended Environment

Be thankful for your house, your family, and your friends. The people and places that make your life simpler or more comfortable in some way. The supermarket, the gas station, the cafes, and the restaurants — the trash collectors, the cab and uber drivers, weather forecasters, physicians, nurses, healers, and holistic practitioners.

Express gratitude for the city and the nation in which you live, the freedom and privileges that are at your disposal.

The physical world around you — the birds you hear outside your window, the flowers, trees, parks, playgrounds, rivers, mountains, oceans, and the fish that swim in them.

Continue to extend your knowledge outward, fostering an appreciation for everything that you can think. You can also feel grateful for the Earth, the Solar system, the Stars, and for Life itself! Gently allow your mind to go over one subject to another while actively disciplining appreciation for all that happens to you.

If you can put the book down, try it now or do this later, try to maintain this state for at least 10 minutes and gradually increase the time.

Consider Increased Happiness

When finished, open your eyes, and take a moment to remember the pleasure that comes with expressing this kind of appreciation. I thank God for this moment of love and gratitude. I am thanking him for every comfort in my life.

It is necessary to pause and remember that tiny, gradual improvements in your everyday life will build-up and strengthen your mental health muscle.

This simple meditation can have a profound effect on your mind and resonance. If you make it a ritual every day, you will find it so much easier to feel more joy and happiness.

And that is significant because to obtain what you want; you must become a vibrational match.

If you want to enjoy more, you need to understand more of what you already have and be grateful for what you want to attain in life.

Gratitude is the fastest way to raise your vibrational frequencies. Your world will transform; it's that simple.

When you practice progressive gratitude like this, you will also find that you will attract more like-minded, hopeful, and happy people in your life.

You will find that things will begin to come to you more effortlessly, and you will naturally feel more motivated to climb the ladder of success.

And not only will it make you feel more joy and satisfaction in life – it will improve your desire to have an impact on the planet and build a positive ripple effect that will inspire others to turn up in the world more positively and happily as well.

CHAPTER 8
MEDITATION FOR SPIRITUAL GROWTH, ENLIGHTENMENT, AND HAPPINESS

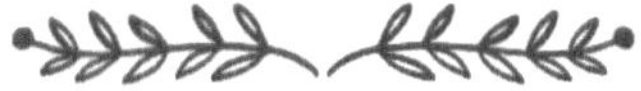

"Spirituality is not adopting more beliefs and assumptions, but uncovering the best in you."

Meditation is a strategy to eliminate yourself from the three-dimensional world and start the correspondence with Heaven's high domains in the Spiritual Unseen World. The reason for meditation is to find our actual selves – a spiritual being living in a physical body and experience genuine bliss by feeling liberated from this material world's limitations.

While we are living in the natural world, we will, in general, overlook that we are spiritual creatures whose genuine home is the Spiritual World. When we become inundated in the third-dimension estimations, our mind gets shady, and our physical body also slowly feels increasingly exhausted. The way to facilitate this exhaustion is to furnish the spirit with an opportunity to restore heaven's light spiritually. To do this, we must detach our three-dimensional consciousness incidentally and, through the right fixation, interface with the Heavenly Realm. The spirit can re-establish its intrinsic energy by getting God's light through proper meditation.

How To Set Up The Mind For Right Meditation

Before entering a meditative state, it is critical to keep our mind tranquil. Suppose we begin rehearsing mental fixation without quieting the mind's vibrations. Before we can experience the spiritual dimension, the entryway to our subliminal should be open, and for this to happen, we need to calm the surface consciousness.

The individual who lives in a decent-hearted way, who endeavors to have great thoughts and carry out beneficial things in their life, can without much of a stretch begin reaching their spiritual guidance when they quiet the surface consciousness. But the individual who has few great thoughts and barely ever tries to carry out beneficial things will go under negative spiritual impacts.

Seeking out the guidance of a spiritual expert is imperative and one you completely trust. Exploration of the Right Mind is an "unquestionable requirement" for the right meditation. Self-reflection rehearsed consistently causes us to keep up the Right Mind as the set up for meditation. Regarding your condition to ponder, it is imperative to pick a peaceful spot where you will not be upset by typical vibrations. Pick a quiet and serene place in your home, or your place of worship are ideal spots to contemplate and ponder to create calm beats, also because they are spiritually protected.

Spiritual Meditation

Do you wish for a sensational change in your body, genuinely, intellectually, and inwardly? At that point, you must back off, feel inward, and become mindful of yourself. It requires an additional push to liberate from the world's frantic energy and tune in to what your body is stating. Put in that extra exertion through spiritual meditation and experience the enchanting contemplation, an encounter that takes you to the profound nature of your identity.

As your genuine self, you can deprive an apparent multitude of recognitions you had about yourself until that point in your life. Simultaneously, you experience delight and harmony. A sentiment of affection and light heats your being.

Spiritual contemplation causes you to understand the eternal truth and let go of all that has occurred and will occur. The present is the place you need to be and discover comfort the need to practice spiritual meditation comes from the inner knowledge of the world-encompassing you.

The Spiritual Meditation Technique

Pick A Comfortable Position

Before you start the training, the most significant viewpoint is to discover a place that you will be comfortable with, including avoiding the city's commotions however much as could be expected, and encircle yourself with greenery and the delicate tweeting of winged creatures. Spiritual meditation can immediately take care of you. To start, be careful about the position you wish to contemplate. Pick a place and post that you are comfortable in but not excessively unwinding, making you virtually drift off into sleep. Sit with your back straight in an easy cross-legged, half-lotus or full lotus, on a gel cushion, or lie down in a corpse pose, if you can stay consciously alert throughout your meditation. The important thing is to set the intention beforehand, so whatever works for your purpose will go with the flow, and if you do fall asleep then know, your physical body needed the rest. At that point, close your eyes delicately.

Experience The Process

When you have the assignment to achieve, what do you typically do? You plan to have the technique in your mind and follow the example deliberately. That is how we are accustomed to doing assignments. We design and execute them in a controlled way. However, this is not the ideal method to manage meditation. Here, it would help if you released it. Release up and let it flow through to its logical end naturally. It would be best if you were an aloof onlooker, permitting the cycle to occur all alone. Try not to bother about hitting the nail on the head or be worried about the result. Allow it to stream in its natural course.

Acknowledge The Thoughts

We experience a daily reality such that sudden spikes in demand for data. You are regularly taken care of with current information as live updates, breaking news, and online media. Subsequently, your mind is continuously buzzing with an unknown substance and your cerebrum's response to it. It is an endless game if you are conscious, and, in any event, it is a severe undertaking to quiet your buzzing mind during sleep.

You frequently respond to each idea and wind up being influenced by it. Indeed, even while you sit to ponder, thoughts will assault you. But the test lies in not reacting to them and permitting them to control you. Let the thoughts leak in like they usually do but hold the desire to respond to them. Let them float away, empowering you to return to your meditation.

Express A Prayer

As you stay here, keeping your thoughts from insulting your quiet self-restraint, pick a prayer in your mind. You can articulate whatever implies something bravo or something that you like. It could be a word or an expression. It could be something identified with wildlife if you are a nature sweetheart or something that satisfies you. It could be a chant, a prayer, or the silent or verbal repetition of the names of God.

Presently, keep your body free and loose. Inhale naturally and gradually. Watch your breath as it goes in and out. Thoughts will intrude on your cycle, but you recognize what to do with them. Return to your body and breathe after each idea or story interferes. At that point, at every exhalation, think about the prayer you picked. Articulate it in your mind each time you inhale out. Utilize devotion to bringing back your regard for watching your breath.

Reflect On Yourself

Direct your concentration toward your body and your mindfulness and presence in the space. Become aware of your environmental factors. See how your body feels. Be mindful of your thoughts and breath. Unwind totally and remain quiet. Open your eyes gradually and sit similarly situated for quite a while. Let the impacts of meditation hit home. Feel it and appreciate the softness your body feels. Consider the whole cycle and how you went about it. Notice how you have gotten less upset than before the meditation. Acknowledge that your response to the revelation was natural.

Interconnected Pathways Of Meditation & Spirituality

Meditation and spirituality are two fascinating words that identify with one another. When you talk about spirituality, it alludes to limitless consciousness in a person. However, this does not imply that spirituality and spiritualism are comparative as spiritualism is a different idea worried about mediums utilized to contact the spirit world.

Spirituality is a similar truth that one understands through the extraordinary spiritual instructors of the World. Instructors in history like the sages and Prophets are, overall, spiritual educators who have all come with the same message, the truth, and "BELIEF" in "ONE GOD" they all guided their nation's supporters to arrive at their boundless consciousness. To them, one's life's objective lies in combining the individual mind to reach limitless consciousness by utilizing spiritual meditation.

When you discuss meditation, it alludes to a type of concentrated reasoning. This full reasoning is not only any type of focused rationale; it is where you need to make your mind concentrate on the wellspring of consciousness found inside yourself. It is not possible short-term; only after persistent and vigorous meditations, you will find that your consciousness is unbounded. Hence, it is just that numerous times, the objective of meditation is "self-acknowledgment."

Recollect that meditation is a tranquil and limitless substance; you cannot seek it out promptly on demand. However, sometimes it is just your fixation. Will you understand that there is bliss waiting for you; and that there is agreement, euphoria, and a mindfulness inside you that is standing by to be recovered and perceived.

Some are trying to get illumination or have a type of spiritual experience, resort to utilizing meditation as a medium or vehicle to arrive at spirituality.

It is possible to become more profound in degrees of mindfulness in your mind-body, and soul through meditation.

You should rehearse seriously with relentless assurance if you need to arrive at your feeling of spirituality through meditation. Spirituality is not something that can be obtained or reached without exertion from your side. Numerous people attempt to evade the countless hindrances that may come their way when looking for improvement through spirituality. Any boundaries in meditation will defeat the purpose of illumination.

Numerous people inquire as to whether there is an alternate route to meditation and spirituality. To arrive at genuine realization through meditation if you initially get the opportunity to arrive at illumination. Besides utilizing meditation, you can accomplish this in a more viable and faster technique by longing for improvement and spirituality. Simultaneously, it is also significant that you stay fair with yourself all through the cycle.

With meditation, it is also possible to arrive at spirituality by "destroying" and "delivering" whatever conscience or personality you have in your energy field through and through. Numerous times, it is this personality or conscience in yourself that may hamper your advancement in meditation.

On arriving at spirituality or enlightenment through meditation, you will, in general, experience a sentiment of kindness, expansion, softness, inward peace, certainty, internal information, energy, and pure love for the Creator and the creation and the self as well. It is also possible for you to build up a profound association with the planet, the universe, and distinct species while encountering a sentiment of lightness, versatility, and internal knowing in yourself.

You can reach or accomplish spirituality with challenging work, assurance, and the correct type of contemplation.

How Meditation Helps You Become More Spiritually Self-Connected In Wisdom

Is it accurate to say that you feel a nudge from your profound inside to become more associated with your spiritual self but continually occupied by the worry in your life? Would you like to be in an arrangement with your actual calling? Would you like to encounter additional significance in your life and increase knowledge from the spiritual aides and educators that come your way? For any of your inquiries, meditation is the appropriate response.

Our Consciousness Is Continually Unfurling In Unobtrusive & Significant Manners

What is preventing you from living in a more illuminated state? It could be a negative idea design. It could be fortuitous. It could be the mounting weight on your plate. Great news. Turning out to be in order and associated with a higher domain of spirituality can be accomplished through the act of meditation. And when you participate in it consistently, you will not merely make an open door for your mind to pick up clarity from the quietness. Still, you will have the option to disengage from your personality and reveal the cover of what is past yourself – and associate with your most elevated self.

We Are Spiritual Beings Having A Physical Experience

When we are associated with our spirituality through meditation, we quit feeling a different being. Meditation allows us to venture outside of our Ego, disengage from the weights, stress, and commitments of our lives, and become aligned with a spot within ourselves that is never without anything that we need. Whatever your spiritual practice, meditation offers a similar advantage to all – a wellspring in a league of its own.

Self-Esteem & Creating Merciful Love For Everyone & Everything

And as the most significant advantage of meditation and spirituality, think about this: as we become more in order and associated with our spiritual self, we become more receptive to our identity and what we must do in this life becoming sincere for giving unconditional love, mercy, and compassion to the creation without any expectations. Need a reason? Attempt meditation for a spiritual reason!

If you are new to meditation as training, you may begin five to fifteen minutes out of each day. It may appear as though nothing is going on from the start, but you will become more comfortable with it eventually. At that point, you will begin to feel the quieting spiritual and enthusiastic advantages of this training. You should expand your meditation to thirty minutes to an hour on more than one occasion per day. Recall that you should not drive results or be restless. However - your meditation needs to advance if you are genuinely going to profit from it. Regardless of whether you miss a day, proceed with your everyday practice like nothing has occurred.

Keep in mind; meditation is a cycle of developing and advancing spiritually and personally. Your strategy and objectives will all vary, and you may need to investigate to discover the appropriate technique for you. However, anybody can profit by including meditation in their day. We are all on a spiritual, mental, and enthusiastic self-development path, and meditation is a magnificent apparatus to assist us with arriving. Whether you decide to work with an educator, use meditation materials like audios, books, and chronicles, or ruminate all alone, it can genuinely help. Accommodating meditation into your daily life is an extraordinary strategy to enable you, to get where you would prefer to be.

CHAPTER 9
BUILD A POSITIVE SPIRIT
AND MINDSET

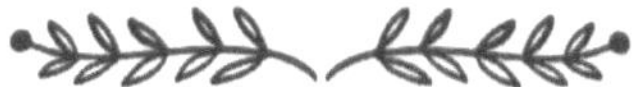

"Change your thoughts and you will change your world."

Have you ever been in that state of mind where you are battling to keep a positive mindset even though everything around you may not feel okay?

Would you be able to figure out how to think positively? You have heard some things about the advantages of positive reasoning. Examination recommends that positive scholars have better pressure adapting abilities, more grounded invulnerability, and a lowered risk of cardiovascular infection. While it's anything but a wellbeing panacea, taking a realistic view instead of ruminating on negative thoughts can profit your general mental prosperity.

It is typical for us to make arrangements and hold desires, but one of the most consistent things in life is frustration. When this happens, we will, in general, become overpowered and debilitated. Lamentably, the more we harp on these negative thoughts, the more we might probably lose all sense of direction in them.

I have considered why we are more disposed to have a negative mentality than a positive one. Why is it that when we invest some extensive energy and exertion getting and applying tips to building up a cheerful and enthusiastic demeanor, one paltry occasion will happen and send us starting over from the beginning? Why is it that this pattern of trouble spins endlessly, and regardless of how enthusiastically we experiment, it appears to be impossible to end it forever? I have understood that it generally comes from our thoughts and feelings. Negative disposition is a result of negative thoughts, arising from negative responses, which results in negative conduct.

So what would you be able to do to turn into an optimistic scholar? A couple of traditional techniques include figuring out how to identify negative thoughts and supplanting these thoughts with more positive ones. While it may require some investment, inevitably, you may find that reasoning positively begins to come all the more naturally.

Positivity As A State Of Mind

Let me tell you a story about a woman who demonstrated happiness and positivity amidst all her hopeless challenges.

A woman who was more than 90 years of age was extraordinary in dressing up well, applying her make-up, and dressing up her hair in wonderful elegant styles.

She and her husband had been married to one another for over 70 years, such a very long time. After her cherished partner's demise, having no children and nobody in the family to care for her, she had to move to a nursing home.

Indeed, even on the day she abandoned her home for good, she dressed up exquisitely and looked beautiful. After showing up at the nursing home, she waited calmly in the entry way for quite a long time before her room was accessible.

At the point when her chaperon came up to advance her towards her room, she gave her attendant a visual portrayal of the small room that she was to possess.

"I love it," The elderly woman said with the excitement of an eight-year-old who had recently been gifted with a puppy.

"Maam, you haven't even seen your room yet... wait until you see it" The attendant said to her. "Indeed, My euphoria has nothing to do with the room," The old woman answered.

"My excitement for the room is not dependent on how beautiful the furniture is or how it's arranged, it depends upon how I organize my mind, happiness is something I have decided before its time. No matter what, I have decided to adore my room, to cherish the people around me, and to adore my life. It is a choice that I make each day, everytime I wake up. Let me tell you something, the best resource we as a whole have, is the ability to choose how we feel."

The elderly woman kept talking as the attendant listened mindfully with her mouth gaped open.

"I can go through my whole day in bed thinking of the agony I am in, grumbling about the parts of my body that presently don't work or I can get up and be grateful for those parts that do move and accomplish my work. Every day is a gift, and as long as my eyes are open, I will keep on zeroing in on today and all the cheerful memories I have put away in my mind, only for this time in my life."

The attendant was astonished by the older woman's positive attitude, whose life from an outside perspective was just loaded with problems and hopelessness.

Given the circumstances, it is certain problems will come. So happiness is a decision we as a whole need to make.

"Contempt" happens naturally "love" is a decision we as a whole need to make.

Being negative happens; consequently, a positive attitude is a decision we need to make.

"Complaining" is certain, but in such a situation, "Gratitude" is a decision we as a whole need to make.

Look at how the woman stayed positive, despite her hopeless condition. Life's happenings are seen by other people differently. It resembles choosing the "half-vacant" or "half-filled" approach. In all actuality, satisfaction is controlled by the position our mind's take on of the situation.

When you are complaining about not having shoes, seeing a person without a foot will comfort the purposeful hardship you have endured. Satisfaction and the ensuing bliss are consistently accessible in our minds, even in the most unfriendly or hostile circumstances. It is possible to discover motivations to have a sentiment of relative prosperity, even in difficulties, from inside our minds, we frequently do the opposite. A considerable lot of us have adapted to the point that in any event, when we have the most evident motivations to feel the delights of life, we search out for issues to justify our staying miserable.

Youth moulding, parental and social impacts make people see life positively or contrarily. Confirmations to this are accessible among different world networks. We discover some of them in a general sense of giddy, some unendingly numb, and some others never-ending in the encounter. Since joy is a mind-work, handling dismay at the degree of the mind, we can yield more successful outcomes. Numerous spiritual masters are regularly equipped for working up positivity among their supporters through proposals and directing. We also realize that therapists impact their customers and change their mindset into positivity, expectation, and resilience.

Positive reasoning is one thing that should be developed amongst kids directly from the earliest starting point, except if the parental and social negativities are handled first, giving mind-care contributions to youngsters won't work appropriately. This requires mindfulness age among guardians, youngsters, and those firmly associated with kids improvement. The educational domain that can do this mindfulness age is Psychology. However, Psychology stays excessively specialized and getting simplified for regular mindfulness soon is far off. This is the idea of preparing mind-care experts with information on rudiments of Psychology and directing aptitudes. When they connect with the concerned people, it might be possible for them to change their mindsets and work on positivity in the public arena.

Spiritual Growth Mindset: The Secret To Manifesting Success

You may have found out about Growth Mindset, yet precisely what is a Spiritual Growth Mindset?

After reflecting, I might want to propose building up a profound development attitude and not only a positive outlook. A profound development mentality would be one that is additionally supporting, mindful, and broad. Let me share a portion of my considerations beneath.

RAS - Set Up A Positive System To Accomplish Your Goals

RAS stands for reticular activating system, an extremely active network within the human brain developed to refine the impressive amount of information. This cell network works similarly to a filter retaining only the important data, which, later, should undergo a stockage process. The conscious mind meets first the tremendous amount of information while the subconscious receives exclusively relevant information. The transition between these two stages is based on a filtering mechanism - reticular activating system. Further on, we will detail the basic criteria or filtering stimuli that activate the RAS:

1. Life-related issues

   RAS sets in motion all inner connections the moment when the human brain comes across vital pieces of information.

2. New relevant content

   The reasoning network is developed to retain and maintain for limited time highly important information.

3. Emotionally relevant information

   There are so many things going on in our lives and around us daily that it is impossible for us to focus on everything; therefore, we need to filter out all the things that are of no importance to us.

The reticular activation system helps us to focus on all those things that we are either thinking about or are important to us and filters out everything else that is of less importance.

Suppose you think about negative things all the time. In that case, the reticular activation system in your brain will find everything that it can, that is related to what you are thinking about that is happening around you and make it crystal clear so that it is brought to your attention.

The beauty of this part of the brain is that if you start to focus on the things in life that you want and not on those things that you do not wish for, you will find that you have everything that you need at your disposal, but because of what you are focusing on, you usually are just filtering it all out. There are so many opportunities that cross our path every day, but we do not notice them because our focus is on other things.

The reticular activation system is similar to a camera in your brain, and it can make things appear more significant than they are. When we focus on the smaller picture, it can sometimes seem dark and dreary. Still, when you start to step back for a moment and look at the picture as a whole, suddenly the whole picture changes entirely and what we thought was happening was only confined to that situation. The reticular activation system is very closely linked to visualization. When you visualize your success clearly and vividly, feeling that success as if it has already been achieved, your brain will start to filter out all the information that does not serve you and bring all the information that ties in with your vision to your attention.

The key to using your reticular activation system to empower you is to make it clear in your mind through visualization, all the things that are important to you, all the feelings that you want to experience, the love, the joy, the happiness, the success. Your whole attitude will start to change, and the people and opportunities that you had unconsciously blocked out will be brought to your attention. You will be able to experience the happiness, success or any other feelings that you are striving for.

Spiritual Growth Mindset: Set The Intention

Another worldly outlook bolsters the expectation to lead a profoundly cognizant life. Since you are arousing in cognizance, you might want to see existence with a profoundly adjusted focal point. Individuals comprehend mentality as an allowance of faith based expectations or disposition. The convictions let you outline the circumstance that you are in. They decide your recognition of how you see things. Regardless of whether you decipher things to be positive or negative, your mentality plays an enormous part.

A profound mentality is not just about having a lot of elevating convictions. Or maybe, it additionally alludes to a lot of profoundly adjusted beliefs that impact your responses and conduct. Your attitude is a mood that encourages you to move towards massive results. Your consciousness of your profound nature outlines your convictions. They direct you regarding settling on conscious decisions that help your development.

Convictions are considerations. At the point when musings become molded and routine, you characterize yourself by them and who you can turn into. The impact you have at the character level. Numerous individuals battle since they neglect to look at the convictions that they had unknowingly made or made previously.

Issues emerge when they relate to mixed-up thoughts. On the off chance that you want to find your actual nature or discover who you indeed are the ("I" or "I am"), you must shed off the layers of misrepresentations. These falsehoods are probably going to keep you from arriving at your most high potential.

Which Mindset Do You Have? Fixed Or Growth Mindset?

In a fixed mindset, you accept that achievement depends on natural capacity, for example, insight, and ability. You consider them to be 'fixed' attributes. Thus, you invest your energy by demonstrating your knowledge or ability as opposed to creating them.

With a fixed mentality, you are slanted to accept that you cannot make progress where you are not keen enough. If you get that you are not brought into the world with the correct qualities or characteristics, you could choose to receive a pessimist demeanor since it is as though there isn't anything that you can do to change your destiny. Accordingly, you limit your learning and become reluctant to put resources into your development.

On the other hand, in a development growth mentality, you accept that achievement depends on challenging work, picking up, preparing, and determination. Regardless of whether you have cerebrums and ability, you comprehend that they are only the beginning stage. You have a 'gradual view' behind your adoration for learning and disposition of versatility.

In a self-development attitude, your attention is less on the result than what can be accomplished by participating in the learning cycle. Similarly comprehend that nobody has ever scaled extraordinary status — not Mozart, Picasso, or Michael Jordan—without long stretches of predictable practice. You appreciate demonstrating achievement so, you can step up your game.

Demonstrating The Success Mindset For Spiritual Growth

Attitude is something that all extraordinary CEOs, practical business visionaries, thought pioneers, and Olympic competitors know. They have attitude immersion mentors, to help them accomplish increasingly elevated discoveries, and they likewise encircle themselves with tutors, coaches, expert companions, and colleagues with a positive development mindset. It's how unattainable ranks are achieved, and new records are broken every other day.

Settling on the decision to view and approach life from a profound edge would include building up an otherworldly outlook. Thus, it is all-encompassing. As I would see it, genuine progress needs to consolidate otherworldliness.

Build up a Spiritual Growth Mindset for Manifesting Success and Abundance.

I have since discovered that building up an inspirational outlook was, not a short-term thing. It takes study, perusing, going to classes, incorporating conviction changes, and updates in energy framework on an on-going premise.

Awaken Your Positive Spirit

So, here comes the inquiry. What do you do when nothing appears to go right? Do you bow your head down and get into "For what reason is this transpiring" attitude? Or then again, do you venture up and take a gander at the splendid side in any event when it is difficult to spot?

An uplifting disposition is an endearing point for me because, for a long time, I lived on the negative side. Did I begin to comprehend the intensity of positive speculation throughout everyday life by encountering agony and vacancy? The best part is, you can do this switch as well.

Here are three different ways you can stir your soul away from any negative setting:

1. *Movement Creates Emotion*

Envision your normal day. You wake up, prepare, and head to work. For the day, you manage a wide range of issues and difficulties. Cut off times for your huge tasks are making up for the lost time, and your mother just called you, crying that her canine is debilitated, and it does not look great. You work your butt off and by 5 pm you are in something that I call fatigue state. Be that as it may, pause, there is a recreation center to hang out today at 7 pm. You previously guaranteed your mates that you would be there, so you appear.

You snatch your headset and step on the running belt while playing your accumulating persuasive discourses. Inside 15 minutes of movement, you are feeling good. Your heartbeat is racing and you begin running quicker. Following 30 minutes of action and extraordinary exercise, the complete depletion is gone, and you feel incredible. Abruptly, the day does not appear to be so awful, and you feel great about yourself. Why? Because movement is medicine.

Each movement brings a sensational feeling. When I feel sick, something I begin to do is exercise, and state "YES" for 60 seconds. I put my hands up like an Olympic Champion who has won the gold medal, as I hop, skip, and jump, I visualize and grin with a happy smile on my face. It looks insane, so, you won't see me doing it, yet the difference in my psychological state occurs in a moment.

2. *Energy Focus*

How about we investigate this situation. At some point, two significant occasions. The first is acceptable. You finally finalized that negotiation with a substantial customer that you were zeroing in on for quite a long time—an incredible achievement. Yet, at that point, you get an email. It's from the vehicle organization where you applied for your fantasy vehicle. Lamentably, your financial assessment is only a couple of numbers underneath their necessary breaking point, so your application is denied. The inquiry is: Which one are you going to zero in on?

The specialty of satisfaction isn't in not having issues or not encountering misfortunes en route. It's about viewpoint and your capacity to zero in on the additions. Life adjusts itself. I can disclose to you at this moment, with substantial certainty, that you won't generally get what you need or when you need it. Life will frequently invite you with re-fights. On the off chance that you have a great glass half full when things don't go your direction, your inspirational demeanor will spare you every single time.

3. *Commitment*

OK, presently, you might be thinking, "What's going on with commitment in this book when we talk about the uplifting demeanor?" I get it, so it allows me to clarify. Commitment has a profound effect on your emotional well-being.

At the point when you give and offer, without a doubt, you will get appreciation from the other individual. It causes you to feel valuable, significant, and appreciative too. Why? Since there comes when you'll perceive every one of those things, you are underestimating while others are kicking the bucket to have or encounter them. That is the reason we will, in general, feel more thankful when we contribute.

Appreciation enacts optimistic feelings and coordinates your emphasis on beneficial things. You give and get simultaneously. I call this a two-fold victory.

An inspirational mentality is both a cliché and a tasteful subject. It gets silly since we hear it always. However, it remains tasteful because it works and unquestionably spares you from living in wretchedness. In any event, when you do not typically get what you need, with a good mind it will feel like you do.

Taking everything into account, building up an inspirational demeanor help you in a significant number of ways than you may understand. When you think positive considerations, you don't permit your brain (cognizant or subliminal) to engage any opposing thoughts or questions.

After you figure out how to think positively, you will see stunning changes surrounding you. Your mind will start to work in a condition of free-streaming feel-great hormones called endorphins, which will cause you to feel lighter and more joyful. You will likewise see a significant lift in certainty and feel more fit for taking on new tasks and difficulties that may have recently been external to your normal range of familiarity.

By diminishing your self-restricting convictions, you will adequately deliver your brakes and experience development like you never envisioned. You can change as long as you can remember just by tackling the intensity of positive reasoning.

CHAPTER 10
CHANGE YOUR STORY, CHANGE YOUR LIFE

"Change will not come if we wait for some other person or some other time. We are the ones we've been waiting for. We are the change that we seek."

Is that true? If you change your attitude, you can transform your life? Indeed, it is correct. And if you anticipate its arrival, there is an extraordinary experience that awaits you.

Pause, an experience? That seems like fun. Indeed, it very well maybe if you know the principles. You see, life itself is a game. A game you have a decent possibility of winning if you recognize what you are doing, get ready and have the apparatuses to help you through the predicament. And beyond any doubt, there will be a predicament. It would help if you are prepared for it.

Mindset is so significant if you are attempting to make changes in your life.

"We can't take care of issues by utilizing similar reasoning we used when we made them." - Albert Einstein

You must accomplish something else if you need it to be different – you can be propelled by what is going on around you, but you need to roll out the improvement yourself, and one thing is without a doubt that will not occur except if you trust it is conceivable. Altering your mindset – transforms you!

Mindset For Change

Quit fearing what could turn out badly and begin thinking about what could go right!

If you are continually fretting about all the manners in which this will not occur for you, at that point, truth be told, you are going to need to surrender at the primary sign that things are not going great. And they will not.

Anything worth having will, in general, be arduous to achieve. Whatever you are endeavoring towards, you will inevitably come against a mass or the like with the best intentions on the planet. Be that people revealing to you it is not possible, or prolonged periods of challenging work wasting your time (apparently), or your niggling self-doubts (because even the most undoubtedly certain among us have those awful days).

You will have days when you want to quit; it is unavoidable. It is how you react to the tall orders nowadays. If you do not begin with a development mindset and the information that each misfortune or even disappointment is a chance to pick up something, you will surrender at the point of the main obstacle.

Self-conviction is EVERYTHING. Honestly, it is SO significant. You must have such a tremendous amount of trust in your capacity to make the life you need that nothing can contain it, that no one can get you down with a very much implied wake-up call. If you can develop that, you will be relentless.

Coaching Yourself Into A Mindset Of Happiness & A Surging Life

Happiness is a central driver that brings motivation and inspiration for all that we do in life. Carry on with that euphoric flooding, and life is entirely out of handle far more often for many individuals. And while being happy 100% of the time may appear ridiculous to certain people, being happy for a sensible measure ought to be accepted as something other than conceivable.

The accomplishment of happiness, most of the time, at that juncture turns into an issue of how? Numerous people consider what things they ought to do and how life lets them down on such a traditional assumption.

So, the inquiry at that point runs into how we can consistently make a decent degree of happiness. And having experienced some genuine difficulties and trained many individuals through truly upsetting circumstances, I can joyfully say, it is simple to make a happy life for yourself.

Happiness, as you are aware, is an emotional state.

In this state, it is never truly subject to the things you do on a physical level. You love doing something, be it yoga, meditation, driving, voyaging, eating, or whatever. The action is independent of the inclination, however.

You relate a movement with an unrelenting passionate reaction and frequently take action to pick up that enthusiastic momentum.

Taming Your Ego to Practice Humility

Everyone has an ego; the test hosts our ego, so it does not improve us. Many individuals, particularly people from special foundations, regularly battle to keep their egos under check.

They believe the World revolves around them. These are the: "do you know who I am?" It is about the pride they have. This ego, pride keeps them from accepting necessary criticism about themselves, and thus they do not develop as people. We have all been there, and we must be honest with ourselves, own up, recognize it, and move over towards humility.

We cannot take objections if we are unwilling to learn from outside sources. We cannot anticipate openings or make them happen if we are opposed to seeing what is before us. We live inside our dream world that we are superior to the following person.

How To Know If You Are Egotistical

There are some indications that the ego is crazy. For instance, do you complain or pick faults frequently? Do you have to criticize things both vast and little to get your fingerprints on a task? That may be a sign you have to take a stride back. I have been there too, and I do not like that part of me when awareness takes over.

If being critical is your trademark, do you wonder why your thoughts are better than everybody else's? I am not alluding to the regular appraisals that administrators and councils need to perform. But when snarky is simply the standard gag. Contending and battling with others does not ordinarily give the ideal outcomes. If you have profitable recommendations, make them consciously.

Bend over backward not to be a know-it-all. Since we cannot – know everything, that is. We can see a lot, be at a specialist level, or even "composed books" on a subject. But it is typically more viable to let another person give us the credit we deserve. We accomplish better when others advertise for us.

When a situation is reversed, how does your ego show itself? Being guarded when scrutinized is amateurish and juvenile. Rather than accusing others, figure out how to tune in and perceive how much they need to contribute. Allow your associates or subordinates to excel in demonstrating that your ego is not obstructing achievement.

Holding feelings of resentment will not go anyplace either. If you intend to keep working with similar people, you truly need to work with people as a team. Get over yourself! I can let you know from my insight: Sooner or later, you will require their assistance.

If you have severed your family ties, your ego will have a tough stretch attempting to go with the flow for mending the broken relations.

When you make sense that you may have been off-base or violated a limit, be happy to apologize. A little humility is consistently welcome if it is earnest. Concede your mix-ups and offer whatever help or backing you can.

Figure out how to let it go.

1. Let us place this. If you need to beat your ego, you must figure out how to let go of specific things:
2. Let go of being annoyed at each easily overlooked detail.
3. Let go of the need to win and be correct always.
4. Let go of the should be predominant.
5. Let go of identifying yourself by your accomplishments and fame.

Additionally, a couple more things:

1. Keep your temper concealed.
2. Keep your comical inclination.
3. Keep your tone respectful.
4. Keep your mind and your ears open.
5. Keep a guard on your mind chatter and think twice before you speak your thoughts.

At the point when we eliminate ego comes sincere and genuine authenticity.

What replaces ego is humility, indeed, rock-hard humility and certainty. While the ego is artificial, humility holds weight.

- Ego is taken. Certainty is earned.
- Ego is self-blessed; its "walk the talk" is artificial.
- Ego is worried about me frequently.
- Humility is worried about serving others unsurpassed.
- Ego says, "see me;" I am better than everyone else.
- Humility says: "it is not about me;" it is about the work to be done. "Let's get the chance to be a team and work together."

You will co-make amicable relations with everybody on the planet, particularly those you love, by giving up the wounded personality.

Here is a delightful Hawaiian Prayer, ***"I am sorry, please forgive me, I love you, thank you."*** Announce it with enthusiasm and sincerity. Use this prayer if you find yourself in any adverse situation for defusing a hostile atmosphere or restoring the fractured personal relationships, even if you are in the right to be defensive.

If your relationships are agitated or aggressive, be the 1st to apologize and see how people in your life react. Become sincere over your lifetime, be selective with your hearing, ask for forgiveness earlier than making matters worse in your life.

How to Change Your Mind-Set For A Happy Successful Life

Being happy and beneficial is something we aspire. Certainly, when asked, "What's your point in life?" a portion of us would reply – to be happy. But on certain days, this "little and unobtrusive" objective is light-years away.

The great and awful news is this – it is all in our minds. In any event, when it appears to be challenging to look on the splendid side of things, it is 100% in our capacity to change how we see life.

Remember Your Blessings

In the 21st century, we have access to more information endeavoring to expand us continually. However, some of the time, we need to acknowledge what we now have, and abruptly a different world will open directly before us.

Changing your mindset to being appreciative is genuinely one of the most remarkable shockers. It might sound too easy to consider being that powerful, but you need to rehearse it consistently and in all that you do.

If you truly set your focus on being thankful, you will quit focusing on little irritations and adverse circumstances. Instead, you will begin to zero in on the beneficial things that have occurred and the exercises you have gained even, from undesirable occasions or experiences.

Start By Doing This Straightforward Exercise Each Night Before You Rest:

Record 7 happy things that happened today: you are grateful for, even little pleasure's like having a heavenly latte in the morning or getting a benevolent grin from an associate or a loved one or making someone smile or sending a silent prayer for happiness to them.

As you practice this procedure (without interferences!) for a little while or months, you will notice to value these little delights of life as of now at the time when you experience them.

Discover Your Purpose

Go through a day alone and ponder what you need to accomplish in this life. This thought can appear to be ambiguous toward the start.

For instance, it is feasible a substantial portion of us would state that we need to be happy and fruitful. But set aside the effort to look further into what these ideas intend for you. Your motivation may be to accomplish something important consistently or improve the world a spot by doing what you love. Your point can be to develop one percent each day, and you will have transformed 365 percent self-transformed in the year that is a giant leap – personally and expertly.

You can likewise set down more solid objectives for yourself. For instance, go throughout the week's end with your family, get advancement, or take an educational journey to an extraordinary land.

For this situation, take up goal-setting specific periods for accomplishing these achievements.

Attain Fulfillment, Happiness & Contentment

Rather than endeavoring to be happy, I look forward to continued fulfillment. Progressively more therapists and scholars are focusing on the fact that happiness is not a result. It is the only way to be successful in every fiber of our being. Every situation is temporary so, make the most out of every moment in your life from now on.

Being happy and peaceful with yourself and others, go live that extraordinary life you aspire, joy is your birthright, live out a blissful, beautiful legacy, believe it, you can be happy and prosperous in both Worlds.

CONCLUSION

Learning how to have the mindset for success, happiness, and inner peace is crucial when you want a prosperous and blissful life. If you have many goals, you want to achieve. Whatever these goals are, the key is to have growth and a positive mindset rather than a negative personality.

Many times, we have self-imposed limits on ourselves without even realizing what we have done. We then carry those limitations around with us for years, even a lifetime. During your infancy, you absorbed many of your beliefs about yourself, the people in your life, and the World. Think about it; what do you believe about your image, physical body, capabilities, and finances? Journal an audit about any areas of your life, and you will have a belief about it. And you have gathered a lifetime of evidence to "prove" your beliefs right.

Taking on a creative philosophy does not make you the Thomas Edison of today; I allow you to look at your World as though you were an architect. You have a new perspective, a new filter to experience life through, a new way of doing things that will render you a different result. Taking on a new mindset is experimental. Despite this, you may find yourself stuck, unable to act as if you are your chosen belief. If you are having trouble taking on your desired attitude, here are few questions to ask yourself:

"What is stopping me?" There may be something real or perceived stopping you from living your chosen impression. Take an honest look at the beliefs that are stopping you.

"What would happen if I took on a different approach" Are there any concerns about your safety while you have this mindset? Explore that, if you are putting yourself in harm's way, reconsider the context of your attitude.

"Have I ever lived this mindset in the past?" Pull from your past. Do you associate this mindset with any negative results from your past? Put aside any judgment and explore your history and identify what happened with the way you speculated.

"What else would I bring into my life if I lived this new way of thinking?" Exploring what changes you could bring into your life will provide you with additional positive motivational leverage.

"If my wife/husband/brother/sister/best friend were here, what might she or he say I am not seeing about living this mindset?" Chasing another perspective will open extra options and solutions.

"How would it feel if I could find a way to live this mindset?" Break out your crystal ball and start seeing a better future. Partner this question with "And how might I find a way to live this mindset?"

And finally, "if I could find a way to live this philosophy anyway, what might I have to do first?" uncover the first step to living the perspective of your choice. Then you can train your wings to fly in formation.

When you take the time to explore the questions, you will uncover your limiting beliefs honestly. You may even show some of your self-sabotaging behaviors, and you will take a giant step towards claiming this angle because now you are aware of what has been holding you back, what could happen if you make this change and start the change process. With this new awareness, you are already living the mindset you have selected.

Happy people see the good rather than the bad in situations and people. If something happens that upsets or irritates you, remind yourself about switching to a more positive frame of mind. Ask yourself what the good things about the situation are and answer with "if this hadn't happened, I wouldn't now be able to..." or "Now that this has occurred, I can do." Stop getting into an entirely negative mindset and stop yourself thinking that the situation that seemed so awful means that nothing good can happen to you from now on. Every moment you can change your mindset to achieve your desired outcome. In reality, there are no problems only solutions!

REFERENCES

1. Maruyama, M. (1980). Mindscapes and Science Theories, Current Anthropology, Vol. 21, No. 5. (Oct., 1980), pp. 589-608

2. Maruyama, M. (1988). Dynamics among Business Practice, Aesthetics, Science, Politics, and Religion. Cultural Dynamics 1988; 1; 309-335

3. Yolles, M.I, Fink, G., 2014, Personality, pathology and mindsets: part 1-3. Vol. 43 n. (1)

4. Sagiv, Lilach; Schwartz, Shalom H. (2007). "Cultural values in organizations: insights for Europe" European Journal of International Management.1 (3): 176. :10.1504/EJIM.2007.014692. ISSN 1751-6757.

5. Yolles, Maurice; Fink, Gerhard (2016-11-20). "Maruyama Mindscapes, Myers-Briggs Type Indicators and Cultural Agency Mindset Types" SSRN 2873082.

6. Yolles, Maurice; Fink, Gerhard (2013). "Exploring Mindset Agency Theory" SSRN 2369874.

7. Dweck, Carol (2006). Mindset: The New Psychology of Success. New York: Ballantine Books. ISBN 978-0-345-47232-8.

8. "Stanford University's Carol Dweck on the Growth Mindset and Education." OneDublin.org. 2012-06-19.

9.   Dweck, Carol S. (September 2010). "Even Geniuses Work Hard" Educational Leadership. 68 (1): 16–20.

10.   Watkins, P. C., Woodward, K., Stone, T., & Kolts, R. L. (2003). GRATITUDE AND HAPPINESS: DEVELOPMENT OF A MEASURE OF GRATITUDE AND RELATIONSHIPS WITH SUBJECTIVE WELL-BEING. Social Behaviour & Personality, 31(5), 431.

11.   Wood, A. M., Joseph, S. & Maltby (2009). Gratitude predicts psychological well-being above the Big Five facets. Archived 2011-09-28 at the Wayback Machine Personality and Individual Differences, 45, 655-660.

12.   Wood, A. M., Joseph, S., & Linley, P. A. (2007). Coping style as a psychological resource of grateful people. Archived 2011-09-28 at the Wayback Machine Journal of Social and Clinical Psychology, 26, 1108–1125.

13.   Wood, A. M., Joseph, S., Lloyd, J, & Atkins, S. (2009). Gratitude influences sleep through the mechanism of pre-sleep cognitions. Archived 2011-09-28 at the Wayback Machine Journal of Psychosomatic Research, 66, 43-48

14.   Anand, P (2016). Happiness Explained. Oxford University Press.

15.   Feldman, Fred (2010). What is This Thing Called Happiness? ISBN 978-0-19-957117-8.

16.   The Stanford Encyclopedia of Philosophy states that "An important project in the philosophy of happiness is simply getting clear on what various writers are talking about." https://plato.stanford.edu/entries/happiness/ Archived 2018-06-11 at the Wayback Machine.

17.   "Two Philosophical Problems in the Study of Happiness." Archived from the original on 2018-10-14. Retrieved 2018-10-13.

18. Smith, Richard (August 2008). "The Long Slide to Happiness." Journal of Philosophy of Education. 42 (3–4): 559–573. doi:10.1111/j.1467-9752.2008.00650. x.

19. Maisel, Eric. Novato, California: New World Library (published 2010). ISBN 9781577318422. Retrieved 19 September 2019.

20. Wilkinson, Tony (2007). The lost art of being happy: spirituality for sceptics. Findhorn Press. ISBN 978-1-84409-116-4.

21. Browner, Matthieu Ricard; translated by Jesse (2003). Happiness: A guide to developing life's most important skill (1st pbk. ed.). New York: Little Brown. ISBN 978-0-316-16725-3.

22. Ellison, Christopher G.; Daisy Fan (Sep 2008). "Daily Spiritual Experiences and Psychological Well-Being among US Adults". Social Indicators Research. 88 (2): 247–71. doi:10.1007/s11205-007-9187-2. JSTOR 27734699. S2CID 1447127

23. Claussen, Geoffrey (2012). "The Practice of Musar" Conservative Judaism. 63 (2): 3–26. doi:10.1353/coj.2012.0002.

24. Pillars of Islam, Oxford Islamic Studies Online

25. Azeemi, K.S., "Muraqaba: The Art and Science of Sufi Meditation". Houston: Plato, 2005. (ISBN 0-9758875-4-8), p. xi

26. Alan Godlas, University of Georgia, Sufism's Many Paths, 2000, University of Georgia Archived 2011-10-16 at the Wayback Machine.

27. Nuh Ha Mim Keller, "How would you respond to the claim that Sufism is Bid'a?", 1995. Fatwa accessible at: Masud.co.uk

28. Zubair Fattani, "The meaning of Tasawwuf," Islamic Academy. Islamicacademy.org

29. Hawting, Gerald R. (2000). The first dynasty of Islam: The Umayyad Caliphate AD 661–750. Routledge. ISBN 978-0-415-24073-4. Google book search.

30. Ahmed Zarruq, Zaineb Istrabadi, Hamza Yusuf Hanson – "The Principles of Sufism."

31. Richardson, W. Mark. Science and the spiritual quest: new essays by leading scientists Psychology Press, 2002 ISBN 0-415-25767-0, 978-0-415-25767-1

32. Giniger, Kenneth Seeman & Templeton, John. Spiritual evolution: scientists discuss their beliefs. Templeton Foundation Press, 1998. ISBN 1-890151-16-5, ISBN 978-1-890151-16-4

33. Elaine Howard Ecklund, Science vs Religion: What Scientists Really Think. Oxford University Press, 2010. ISBN 978-0-19-539298-2

34. Dalai Lama, The universe in a single atom: the convergence of science and spirituality. Broadway Books, 2006. ISBN 0-7679-2081-3.

35. Capra, Fritjof (1975). The Tao of Physics: an exploration of the parallels between modern physics and Eastern mysticism (1991 3rd ed.). Boston: Shambhala Publications. ISBN 978-0-87773-594-6.

36. Laszlo, Ervin, "CosMos:A Co-creator's Guide to the Whole World" Hay House, Inc, 2008, ISBN 1-4019-1891-3, pp. 53–58

37. D. Bhawuk (2011), Spirituality and Cultural Psychology, in Anthony Marsella (Series Editor), International and Cultural Psychology, Springer New York, ISBN 978-1-4419-8109-7, pp. 93–140.

38. McCormick, Donald W. (1994). "Spirituality and Management" Journal of Managerial Psychology. 9 (6): 5–8. doi:10.1108/02683949410070142.

39. Macrae, Janet (1995). "Nightingale's spiritual philosophy and its significance for modern nursing" Journal of Nursing Scholarship. 27 (1): 8–10. doi:10.1111/j.1547-5069. 1995.tb00806. x. PMID 7721325.

40. MARIFUL QURAN English translation and commentary. "The Explanation, of the HOLY QURAN" by Mufti Muhammad Shafi. Usman Pervez education. Search Google Play.

41. Nur ul Ilm Academy for Sacred Learning and Spiritual Development. The Light of Knowledge. Shaykh Mufti Tauqeer.

ABOUT THE AUTHOR

SARAH JAMES

Sarah is a certified beauty therapist and a holistic hatha yoga specialist. She inspires her readers through her books and writings from her wealth of experience in life.

Sarah is committed to service and sharing her wisdom and knowledge for attaining inner peace, the tranquility of the heart, personal transformation, character development, mindset, holistic wellness, meditation, spirituality, happiness, and living a life of beauty, grace, and purpose.

Sarah is inspired by legendary mentors such as Louise L Hay, Dr. Wayne Dyer, Deepak Chopra, Eckhart Tolle, and Tony Robbins since her early 20's.

She is passionate about attaining self-purification to reach spiritual heights and live a God-conscious life.

Sarah performs her daily rituals of prayers and meditation, experiencing a calm and serene lifestyle.

She loves to cook healthy, delicious meals to break her intermittent fasting. For well-being and exercises to stay lean and fit, you will find her practicing Pranayama, Yoga, Pilates, Qigong, and other Holistic routines.

Sarah likes to maintain an optimistic expression in life, expanding her mindset and spiritual path, accomplishing what she encourages in her writings.

THANK YOU

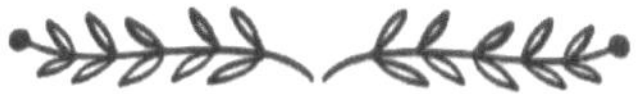

Thank you for purchasing this eBook, paperback, and audiobook.

I hope "The Mind Reset" will help you (Reset Your Mindset, Enhance Your Happiness, Inner Peace & Grace In Your Life).

The next step is to use the guidance in the book to guarantee your success and provide integrity in your life.

Now, please do share the wisdom in this book with your loved ones, family, friends, and associates.

If you enjoyed this book and found it beneficial, I would love your support, and I hope you will be kind enough to post a review for this book.

I will be delighted to hear from you, even if you have feedback, which will help ensure that I improve this book and others in the future.

To leave your Amazon review or go to my book listing or follow the Author, please click the links below.

https://www.amazon.com/review/create-review?&asin=B08VFC2YGM

https://www.amazon.co.uk/review/create-review?&asin=B08VFC2YGM

https://mybook.to/THEMINDRESET

https://author.to/sarahjames

I want to let you know your review is significant to me; it will help secure this book's reach and positively impact many people's lives.

Thank you for your time and support. All the best!

www.ingramcontent.com/pod-product-compliance
Lightning Source LLC
Chambersburg PA
CBHW051055250726
48656CB00001B/314